FACING
OVERWEIGHT
and OBESITY

A Complete Guide for Children and Adults

EDITORS

Fatima Cody Stanford, MD, MPH, MPA

Jonathan R. Stevens, MD, MPH

Theodore A. Stern, MD

FACING
OVERWEIGHT
and OBESITY

A Complete Guide for Children and Adults

Facing Overweight and Obesity – A Complete Guide for Children and Adults

ISBN-13: 978-0-9991483-5-8 (Print)
ISBN-13: 978-0-9991483-6-5 (Ebook)

Book Production: Dianne Russell, Octal Productions, LLC
Copyeditor: Bob Russell, Octal Publishing, LLC
Cover Design: Falcone Creative Design, LLC
Book Design: Dianne Russell, Octal Productions, LLC
Printing and Binding: RP Graphics
Production Managers: Jane Pimental and Grace Shanks, MGH Psychiatry Academy
This book is printed on acid-free paper.

About the Editors

 Fatima Cody Stanford, MD, MPH, MPA, FAAP, FACP, FTOS, Dr. Stanford is an obesity medicine physician at Massachusetts General Hospital (MGH)/Harvard Medical School (HMS). Dr. Stanford received her BS and MPH from Emory University as a MLK Scholar, her MD from the Medical College of Georgia School of Medicine as a Stoney Scholar, and her MPA from the Harvard Kennedy School of Government as a Zuckerman Fellow in the Harvard Center for Public Leadership. She completed her Obesity Medicine & Nutrition Fellowship at MGH/HMS after completing her internal medicine and pediatrics residency at the University of South Carolina. She has served as a health communications fellow at the Centers for Disease Control and Prevention and as a behavioral sciences intern at the American Cancer Society. Upon completion of her MPH, she received the Gold Congressional Award, the highest honor that Congress bestows upon America's youth. Dr. Stanford has completed a medicine and media internship at the Discovery Channel. An American Medical Association (AMA) Foundation Leadership Award recipient in 2005, an AMA Paul Ambrose Award for national leadership among resident physicians in 2009, she was selected for the AMA Inspirational Physician Award in 2015. The American College of Physicians (ACP) selected her as the 2013 recipient of the Joseph E. Johnson Leadership Award and the Massachusetts ACP selected her for the Young Leadership Award in 2015. She is the 2017 recipient of the Harvard Medical School Amos Diversity Award and Massachusetts Medical Society Award for Women's Health.

Jonathan R. Stevens, MD, MPH, is the Chief of Outpatient Services and Child & Adolescent Psychiatry at the Menninger Clinic and an Assistant Professor of Psychiatry and Behavioral Sciences at the Baylor College of Medicine in Houston, Texas. He has trained in both adult and child psychiatry and conducts research on the metabolic side effects of psychiatric medications to identify best practices. As the founder of Menninger's existing outpatient services division, he has led the expansion of unique and personalized services for individuals seeking world-class mental health care. He serves as principal investigator for *BridgeUp at Menninger*, a major initiative to improve the mental health and well-being of disadvantaged youth in Houston. He is the author of scores of articles and book chapters on psychopharmacology and on topics at the intersection of medicine and psychiatry.

Theodore A. Stern, MD is the Ned H. Cassem Professor of Psychiatry in the field of Psychosomatic Medicine/Consultation, Harvard Medical School and Chief Emeritus of the Avery D. Weisman Psychiatry Consultation Service at the Massachusetts General Hospital in Boston, Massachusetts. Dr. Stern has written more than 450 scientific articles and book chapters and edited more than 25 books, including the *Massachusetts General Hospital Handbook of General Hospital Psychiatry* (4/e-7/e), *Massachusetts General Hospital Comprehensive Clinical Psychiatry* (1/e, 2/e), *Massachusetts General Hospital Guide to Primary Care Psychiatry* (1/e, 2/e), *Massachusetts General Hospital Psychiatry Update and Board Preparation*, (1/e-4/e), *Facing Cancer, Facing Diabetes*, and *Facing Heart Disease*. He is also the Editor-in-Chief of *Psychosomatics*.

I would like to dedicate this book to the countless pediatric and adult patients who have taught me about their struggles with obesity. I work tirelessly to address this disease because you drive me to do so.

Fatima Cody Stanford, MD, MPH, MPA, FAAP, FACP, FTOS

To Nicole and our wonderful children Julian, Elliott, and Victoria.

JRS

To our patients, our families, our students, our colleagues, and our mentors. . .

TAS

Acknowledgments

OUR THANKS

This book would not have come into being if not for our patients. They expressed to us their need for a guide to the experience of having heart disease and were so generous in including us in their day-to-day triumphs and struggles. We hope that through this book we were able to fulfill that goal and repay their faith and trust in us.

Without the contributions of so many physicians and related health-care professionals, this book would never have been completed. We thank our contributors for their thoughtfulness and gifted writing as well as their tolerance of our deadlines and edits. We also thank our teachers and mentors for imbuing in us a sense of responsibility to educate, to write with rigor, and, most important, to provide exceptional care to our patients.

At the Massachusetts General Hospital Psychiatry Academy, we thank Grace Shanks and Jane Pimental, our production managers, for their assistance and support. At Octal Publishing, LLC, our thanks go to Bob Russell for his yeoman's efforts related to copyediting, and to Dianne Russell at Octal Productions, LLC for overseeing the production of this book, with grace and style.

FCS
JRS
TAS

TABLE OF CONTENTS

CHAPTER 9
What Lifestyle Changes Can I Make to Address My Obesity?...................... 103
Kim George, MS, RD, LD

CHAPTER 10
Weight-Loss Programs 119
Kim George, MS, RD, LD

CHAPTER 17
Where Can I Turn for Additional Information on Obesity and 205
Its Treatment?
Slyvia Gonsahn-Bollie, MD

GLOSSARY

REFERENCES

INDEX

CONTRIBUTORS

Slyvia Gonsahn-Bollie, MD
Bon Secours, Richmond, Virginia; St. Mary's Hospital, Internal Medicine and Obesity Medicine

Karen J. Campoverde Reyes, MD
Neuroendocrine Unit, Massachusetts General Hospital; Liver Research Center, Beth Israel Deaconess Medical Center, Harvard Medical School, Boston, Massachusetts

Kim George, MS, RD, LD
Massena VA Community-Based Outpatient Clinic, Massena, New York

Sherry Grogan, APRN, PMHNP-BC
The Menninger Clinic, Houston, Texas

Elizabeth Hartwig, BA
The Menninger Clinic, Houston, Texas

Ethan Lazarus, MD, FOMA
Obesity Medicine Physician, Director of Clinical Nutrition Center, Denver, Colorado

Sonali Malhotra, MD
Pediatric Endocrinologist, Massachusetts General Hospital, Boston, Massachusetts; Instructor of Pediatrics, Harvard Medical School

Megan Kale Morcomb, LCSW
Director, Outpatient Assessments, The Menninger Clinic, Houston, Texas

Carl Palad, BS
Medical Student, New York Medical College, Valhalla, NY

Michelle A. Patriquin, PhD
Director, Research Operations, The Menninger Clinic; Assistant Professor of Psychiatry and Behavioral Sciences, Baylor College of Medicine, Houston, Texas

Ajay Shah, MD
Assistant Professor of Child and Adolescent Psychiatry, Texas Children's Hospital, Baylor College of Medicine, Houston, Texas

Rajavi Shah, MD
Assistant Professor of Internal Medicine, US Department of Veterans Affairs, Baylor College of Medicine, Houston, Texas

Juliana Simonetti, MD
University of Utah School of Medicine, Salt Lake City, Utah; Bariatric Medicine Program Director; Co-Director Comprehensive Weight Management Center; Internal Medicine – Assistant Professor (Clinical); Surgery – Adjunct Assistant Professor

Vibha Singhal, MD
Pediatric Endocrinologist, Neuroendocrine Division, MGH Weight Center, Massachusetts General Hospital, Boston, Massachusetts; Instructor of Pediatrics, Harvard Medical School

Fatima Cody Stanford, MD, MPH, MPA, FAAP, FACP, FTOS
Obesity Medicine Physician, MGH Weight Center, Affiliated Faculty Mongan Institute of Health Policy, Associate MGH Disparities Solutions Center, MGH Midlife Women's Center Executive Member; Instructor of Medicine and Pediatrics, Harvard Medical School, Boston, Massachusetts; Executive Committee Member, Nutrition Obesity Research Center (NORCH)

Theodore A. Stern, MD
Chief Emeritus of the Avery D. Weisman Psychiatry Consultation Service, Director of the Thomas P. Hackett Center for Scholarship in Psychosomatic Medicine, and Director of the Office for Clinical Careers, Massachusetts General Hospital; Ned H. Cassem Professor of Psychiatry in the field of Psychosomatic Medicine/Consultation, Harvard Medical School, Boston, Massachusetts

Jonathan R. Stevens, MD, MPH
Chief of Child & Adolescent Psychiatry, Chief of Outpatient Services, The Menninger Clinic; Assistant Professor of Psychiatry and Behavioral Sciences, Baylor College of Medicine, Houston, Texas

Alexander Toth, BA
Clinical Research Coordinator, Laura and Isaac Perlmutter Cancer Center, New York University Langone Medical Center, New York, NY

Humsini Viswanath, BA, MPH
Medical Student, Texas A & M Health Science Center, College Station, Texas

Amy Vyas, MD
The Menninger Clinic; Assistant Professor of Psychiatry and Behavioral Sciences, Baylor College of Medicine, Houston, Texas

Tiffani Bell Washington, MD
Assistant Professor, Psychiatry and Behavioral Medicine, Wake Forest School of Medicine, Winston-Salem, North Carolina

FOREWORD

The Best Information Source in the Battle Against Obesity

Facing Overweight and Obesity is for anyone whose life is affected by this problem. Written by leading physicians in their fields, *Facing Overweight and Obesity* combines top-tier medical information and compassionate counsel on having excess weight with a caring approach to the emotional aspects of living with weight-related conditions. This book provides easily readable and trustworthy information, divided into chapters that ask and answer pertinent questions about being overweight and its medical, surgical, and psychiatric care. A glossary of terms is provided along with tables designed to educate the reader (e.g., about nutrition, diet, exercise, risk-reduction); on-line resources and references are also provided.

PREFACE

Facing overweight and obesity can be hard. Although there are myriad causes for excess weight, and a variety of strategies to lose weight and to maintain that weight loss, this book aims to answer the most common questions asked by people who are facing overweight and obesity. What should I eat? How much should I exercise? What medicines should I take? Should I consider weight-loss surgery? What can my family members do? This book responds to these and other questions.

Not everyone with overweight or obesity experiences it in the same way. Some people cope well, while others develop dread complications (e.g., heart attacks, strokes, diabetes, depression).

Written by experts in endocrinology, psychiatry, and internal medicine, this book addresses medical, emotional, and social aspects of facing overweight and obesity, and answers the questions people affected by overweight and obesity most commonly ask. Since changing dietary and exercise habits is often essential, weight loss usually becomes a family affair. We also discuss how caregivers can learn to face overweight and obesity. Finally, we have provided a glossary of terms (to help you understand the terminology used by medical personnel, and in printed materials) and have provided you with references and resources; these will go a long way toward gaining mastery of interventions for overweight and obesity.

Although this book can be read straight through, from beginning to end, it will work just as well if you prefer to jump from section to section. Feel free to turn to the chapter that interests you most. Your questions will likely change over time, so *Facing Overweight and Obesity* will remain a useful resource. Above all, we think that this book will provide answers to your most pressing questions about how to face overweight and obesity, helping to prepare you and your family for how to live well with these conditions.

FCS
JRS
TAS

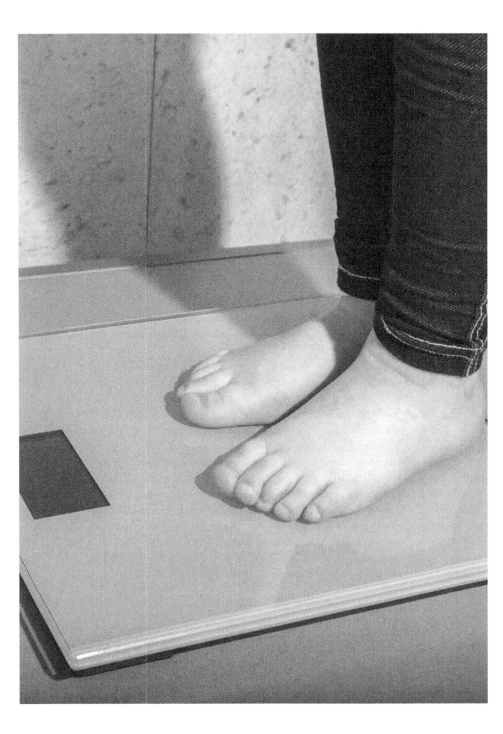

WHAT IS OBESITY?

Sonali Malhotra, MD

In This Chapter

- What Is Obesity?
- How Common Is Obesity?
- Do I Weigh Too Much?
- Why Do I Continue to Gain Weight?
- Why Do I Have Trouble Losing Weight?
- Can I Lose Weight?
- Can Obesity Be Prevented?
- How Does My Body Process and Store Fat?
- Where on My Body Is Fat Likely to Develop?
- How Does Being Overweight Jeopardize My Health and Well-Being?
- Is Obesity Inherited?
- Am I More Likely to Gain Weight as I Age?
- What Can I Do About My Excess Weight?

What Is Obesity?

When your body carries more fat than is defined as healthy for your age and sex, you are said to meet criteria the for *obesity*. In simple terms, obesity occurs when there is an abnormal or excess amount of *body fat*, which is known as *adipose tissue*.

A fat cell is an endocrine cell (a hormone-producing part of your body), and adipose tissue is an *endocrine organ*. Detailed scientific research has demonstrated that this extra fat in the body produces several "bad chemicals," known as *metabolites* or *cytokines*, which have negative influences on health and that ultimately lead to multiple medical problems. Fat produces *inflammation* (i.e., a fundamental way in which your body reacts to infection, irritation, or any other form of injury), which reinforces the fact that this extra adipose tissue in the body causes various disease processes. Excessive fat can eventually lead to your body becoming resistant to a hormone called *insulin*, which tries to keep your blood sugar (*glucose*) in a normal range and ultimately paves the way for development of *type 2 diabetes*.

How Common Is Obesity?

Obesity is one of the most universal chronic diseases. However, there is a pressing need for new guidelines for its medical prevention and treatment.

According to the 14th Annual *State of Obesity: Better Policies for a Healthier America* report from the Trust for America's Health (TFAH) and the Robert Wood Johnson Foundation (RWJF), roughly one in three Americans battle with obesity.

This year, obesity rates among adults topped 35% in five states in the United States (West Virginia led the way at 37.7% followed by Mississippi, 37.3%; Alabama and Arkansas, 35.7%; and Louisiana 35.5%), 30% in 25 states, and 25% in 46 states (California, 25%; Hawaii, 23.8%; Massachusetts, 23.6%; Washington, DC, 22.6%; and Colorado, 22.3% had the lowest rates). This is a substantial increase from the year 2000, when no state exceeded 25% (Fryar et al, 2017). (http://healthyamericans.org/assets/files/TFAH-2017-ObesityReport-FINAL.pdf)

With regard to rates of obesity in children, childhood obesity rates hover around 17%, with nearly one-third (31.3%) of children ages 10 to 17 being overweight or obese. Among high school students, 13.9% are obese. These statistics mean that more than 100 million people in the United States are directly affected by the obesity epidemic, and even more struggle with their weight. These statistics imply that if you look around your workplace and your home, you will see the dramatic impact of the obesity epidemic.

Do I Weigh Too Much?

You can calculate whether you meet the criteria for overweight or obesity by using a simple mathematical formula involving height and weight; it is called the *Body Mass Index* (BMI). The numbers derived from this calculation will help you to categorize your weight, as described in just a moment.

First calculate your BMI by dividing your body weight (in kilograms) by your height (in meters squared [(weight [kg]/height [m]^2 = BMI]) or by using the conversion with pounds (lbs) and inches (in) [Weight (lbs) ÷ height (in)^2] × 704.5 = BMI (https://www.nhlbi.nih.gov/health/educational/lose_wt/BMI/bmicalc.htm).

It is important to remember that this number can be misleading; it can place some people (e.g., those who are very muscular or who are pregnant or lactating) in a category that does not accurately reflect their disease state.

The BMI cutoffs are as follows:

- Below 18.5: Underweight
- 18.5–24.9: Normal weight
- 24.5–29.9: Overweight
- 30 and above: Mild to moderate obesity
- 40 and above: Severe or extreme obesity

If your BMI falls between 18.5 and 24.9, you are considered to have a normal weight. However, if your BMI is equal to or greater than 30, you have obesity (Duerenberg et al, 1991).

BMI is the most commonly used tool to assess someone's weight status, and this is what your doctor will commonly use, as well. However, other indicators of excess fat tissue, such as waist circumference, waist-to-hip ratio, and other measures are also used. Waist circumference is used to determine the fat content around your waistline. An excess of *abdominal fat* or "belly fat" is considered a predictor of *risk factors*, such as a predisposition to heart disease and *type 2 diabetes*.

Now, let's talk about how to measure your waist circumference.

1. First, remove any clothing from your waistline.

2. Stand with your feet shoulders' width apart, and make sure to keep your back straight.

3.   Locate the top of your hipbone. This is the part of the hipbone at the side of the waist, not at the front of your body. Use the area between the thumb and index finger to feel for the hip bone at the side of your waist.

4.   Align the bottom edge of the measuring tape with the top of your hipbone. Wrap the tape measure all the way around your waist. Ensure that the tape measure is parallel (even) with the floor and is not twisted.

5.   Take two normal breaths, and as you exhale the second breath, tighten the tape measure so that it is snug, but not digging into the skin.

6.   Take the measure of your waist.

Now, all of these steps might seem very complicated. A very easy and accurate way to measure waist circumference is to take the measurement at the belly button or navel. This location often captures the widest circumference, and it is directly related to your risk of metabolic diseases, such as type 2 diabetes and heart disease.

The number obtained is your waist circumference. Men with a waist measurement greater than or equal to 40 inches (102 cm) are at risk for multiple health-related problems. Women with a waist measurement of greater than or equal to 35 inches (88 cm) are also at risk for these disorders (Jensen et al, 2014).

Why Do I Continue to Gain Weight?

Your body sets its own target, or *set point*, for fat (Schwartz et al, 2000). Fat is our body's fuel supply, the body's gas tank. There are complex signals and mechanisms that regulate the amount of fat in your "tank." Unfortunately, we do not have complete control of the amount of fat in our tank, and there is a common belief in our society that we are able to voluntarily control the balance of fat in our body by counting calories and burning them with exercise. This is far from true. The body's fat mass goal is determined by a variety of factors, including our genetics, age, race/ethnicity, and environment. The body's fat mass is strongly protected. That is why when someone loses weight by reducing calorie intake, they almost always gain it back (eventually); the body fights to return to its set point—the weight it wants to be at (even if we want it to be otherwise).

Why Do I Have Trouble Losing Weight?

Many people still believe that obesity is caused simply by eating too many calories and exercising too little. Unfortunately, that's a mistaken belief. How the body regulates weight is similar to how it regulates your water balance. If you need water, your brain makes you thirsty, and you drink. If you drink more than you need, your body gets rid of the excess water. It's the same with calories and body fat. You can control it for a short time by eating less, and you might lose weight. But if all you do is eat less, your body will eventually fight back. You'll stop losing weight and ultimately your body will push you to regain all of what you have lost. The same principle allows your body to have a certain set point for fat content; it fights to stay there. It is very frustrating!

Can I Lose Weight?

The first step in weight loss is identifying the key contributing factors that are involved in causing obesity, which varies from person to person. There is not a "one size fits all" approach. The reason behind this is that there are many types of obesity and, as a result, it is necessary to try multiple therapies and combinations of therapies to help different people achieve a healthy weight. Dietary changes might work well for one person, whereas another person might lose weight by improving their sleep habits. We should not expect that there's a simple solution for how you can achieve and maintain a healthy weight. It is critical to understand that obesity is caused by varied biological and *physiological* disruptions in different people, and it is important to match every person to their ideal weight with an individualized treatment approach through exposure to several different methods. Through this strategy, you are most likely to achieve beneficial results and to lose weight. Although interventions (such as engaging in consistent exercise, eating a high-quality diet, practicing stress reduction, and developing good sleep patterns) are at the cornerstone of efforts to achieve and maintain a healthy weight, other individuals might need more invasive interventions (such as medical and surgical interventions) to achieve weight loss. There are multiple medical options available for the treatment of obesity (Apovian et al, 2015). You should talk to your doctor about an appropriate referral to a practitioner trained in obesity medicine, who will complete an interview and a physical examination to decide on the best line of treatment for you.

In conclusion, because obesity is a complex disease, it often needs multiple methods to achieve the desired result of weight loss.

Can Obesity Be Prevented?

Considering the current obesity epidemic, policy makers and national agencies are evaluating various methods and designing programs to help build an environment that can support a healthy lifestyle and ultimately prevent obesity. However, considering the complex and multidimensional etiologies of obesity, it remains a public-health problem.

From an individual perspective, incorporating healthy eating habits (such as eating more fruits, vegetables, and whole grains, and by avoiding processed foods, by cooking meals at home, and by finding healthy recipes) is certainly helpful. Regular physical activity is vital for your overall health and well-being. The amount of exercise needed depends on your age. Most adults need at least 2 hours and 30 minutes (150 minutes) of moderately intense aerobic activity (e.g., brisk walking) every week and muscle-strengthening exercises that work all major muscle groups (legs, hips, back, abdomen, chest, shoulders, and arms) on two or more days per week (WHO, 2004). The exercise doesn't need to be planned. You can find your own ways to incorporate exercise into work (such as taking small breaks for a brief walk, stretching near your computer desk, parking far from the main building so that you get in more steps into your daily step count [approximately 10,000 steps are our daily target]). It is important for you to adopt some consistent form of exercise *that you enjoy* (such as dancing, walking with friends, playing a game). Find what works for you!

Apart from this, avoiding and finding ways to relieve stress, which is part of our modern lives, plays an immensely important part in achieving and maintaining a healthy weight. In addition, it is important to get an adequate amount of sleep, typically 7 to 8 hours for most adults.

How Does My Body Process and Store Fat?

Regulation of body weight and fat tissue appears to be coordinated primarily by our brains. A small area within our brain called the *hypothalamus* receives information from a variety of sources in our body. A hormone, called *leptin*, provides information to the brain about the body's energy stores (Friedman and Halaas,1998). Signals also reach the brain from other organs of your body, such as the *pancreas* and the *liver*, which give information about the energy demands and nutrients availability for the resting energy expenditure and communicates this information to the brain. In terms of food intake, signals about the type, smell, taste, and texture of food are sent to the higher brain centers; these signals along with the others from various organs direct you to start or to stop eating. Overall, the hypothalamus integrates and orchestrates this mass of information and works to achieve a fat set point, which it views as normal for one's body. The storage of fat happens in alignment with this principle, with a constant need to maintain and to achieve that physiological set point.

Where on My Body Is Fat Likely to Develop?

There are different kinds of fat in our body: brown, white, subcutaneous (mostly concentrated in your hips, butt, and thighs), and visceral (mostly in your mid-section). Depending on your gender, race, age, and ethnicity, you might have a predisposition to accumulate different kinds of fat in various parts of your body.

For example, women tend to accumulate more fat around their hips and thighs, whereas men are likely to accumulate it around their bellies (so-called *abdominal fat*). Abdominal fat conveys a greater health risk than does hip or thigh fat. This translates to a greater impact on *insulin resistance*, which increases the risk of diabetes, increases your total cholesterol levels, and predisposes you to an increased risk of *stroke* and heart disease (Schneider et al, 2010).

How Does Being Overweight Jeopardize My Health and Well-Being?

Obesity is now known to have caused or exacerbated more than 40 distinct disorders that lead to poor health and an overall decreased quality of life (Cummings et al, 2002). The medical complications (or *co-morbidities*) range from metabolic problems (such as type 2 diabetes mellitus, high *cholesterol* levels), to high blood pressure, *gallstones*, *fatty liver disease*, *pancreatitis*, *obstructive sleep apnea*, and even reproductive dysfunction. Other diseases that are often associated with obesity include *stress incontinence* (an inability to control your urination), increased pressure within your brain (*idiopathic intracranial hypertension*), which leads to headaches, degenerative joint disease (also known as arthritis), and vertebral disc disease. Scientific research has also provided evidence of a strong association between obesity and many cancers.

Is Obesity Inherited?

So far, we have learned that obesity is a complex condition that results from multiple interactions with *hereditary* and *environmental factors*. It is now well established that different forms of obesity tend to concentrate within families. Obesity risk is two to eight times greater for someone with a family history, as opposed to a person with no family history of obesity; there is an even higher risk observed in those with severe obesity (Zlot et al, 2007).

Studies on twins have compared those who were raised together to those who were raised in a different environment; these investigators have affirmed that genetic influences on BMI are substantial (Stunkard et al, 1990).

There are other rare causes of genetic obesity in which a single gene is affected and leads to more severe forms of obesity; these forms of obesity are seen most often in early childhood. In summary, in most cases, genetic variation influences a person's predisposition for developing obesity, but environmental and psychological factors contribute significantly to the manifestation. Our understanding of how *genes* that contribute to weight and to energy regulation continues to advance rapidly.

Am I More Likely to Gain Weight as I Age?

Aging is characterized by changes in body composition. Imaging studies demonstrate that as we age, subcutaneous fat (the fat below the skin) decreases and the visceral fat (fat in the abdominal region) increases. Visceral fat is not a good thing to have, as we have discussed previously. It is associated with systemic inflammation, and it continues to increase the risk for *coronary artery disease*, *stroke*, and death. Another important age-related change along with altered body composition is loss of muscle mass. Muscle helps us maintain a high metabolic rate and an increased resting energy expenditure. Therefore, its loss is associated with a reduction in the total energy expenditure. The altered body composition and loss of muscle mass leads to fat gain.

Both increases in *visceral fat* and decreases in muscle mass are linked to a loss of sensitivity to insulin. The lower the sensitivity to insulin, the more the body secretes insulin. This metabolic hormone causes a torrent of problems, given that it's a storage hormone. It helps to increase the uptake of glucose and fat production while decreasing the burning of fat and stored glucose (*glycogen*).

What Can I Do About My Excess Weight?

There are multiple effective treatment options available to lose weight. To decide which type of treatment will be best suited for your needs, you will need a comprehensive evaluation completed by a physician trained in *obesity medicine*. In addition, consultation with a *nutritionist* as well as a *psychologist* is also of vital importance. After you have obtained a thorough evaluation, which can include blood testing, your doctor and the entire team will decide on a management plan with you.

The various treatment options available include behavioral, medical, and surgical options. Behavioral treatment involves making lifestyle modifications (such as making better food choices, incorporating more hours of exercise in your routine, and maintaining a healthy and consistent sleep schedule).

If your doctor thinks that making lifestyle modifications will not be helpful by themselves (which is often related to a history of consistent lifestyle changes, severe obesity, or moderate obesity with many obesity co-morbidities (e.g., high blood pressure, type 2 diabetes, obstructive sleep apnea), he or she might choose to prescribe a medicine. There are various weight-loss medicines available that might be used to lose weight; however, only a doctor may prescribe these for you. After you start on a medication, you need to be followed to assess the benefits and side effects of the medicine. These medications are prescribed for long-term use, as discontinuing these medications often leads to weight gain.

If you are suffering from severe obesity, your obesity-medicine doctor might recommend *weight-loss surgery*, which is also known as *bariatric surgery*. Several weight-loss operations have been devised over the past 40 to 50 years. The operations performed by such surgeons includes *Roux-en-Y gastric bypass*, *gastric banding* (adjustable or non-adjustable), *sleeve gastrectomy*, *biliopancreatic diversion*, or *duodenal switch*. If surgery is the preferred therapy for you, this will be a joint decision made by you and your medical team; your surgeon will inform you about the various forms of surgery best suited for your needs. To date, surgery is the most effective treatment for those with severe obesity. Overall, it is important to utilize the appropriate tools for the best outcomes in obesity treatment.

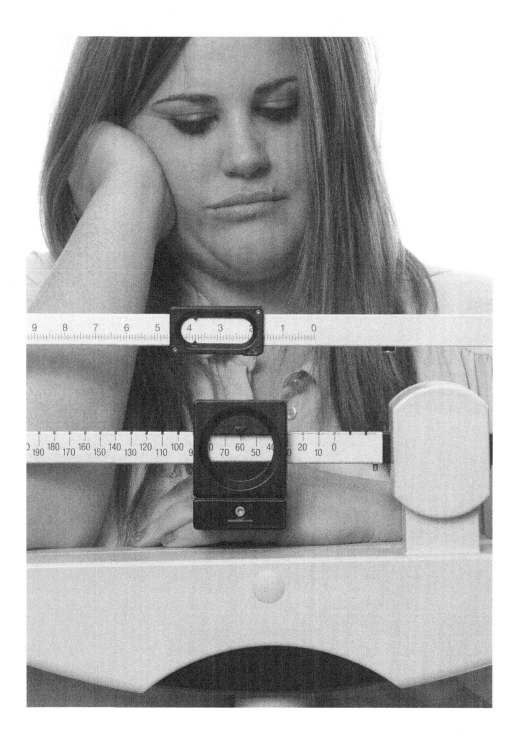

ARE MY FEELINGS ABOUT BEING OVERWEIGHT NORMAL?

Elizabeth Hartwig BA; Humsini Viswanath BA, MPH; and
Michelle A. Patriquin, PhD

CHAPTER

In This Chapter

- Is There a Normal Way to Feel About Having Excess Weight?

- How Am I Likely to React When Others Tell Me That I Should Lose Weight?

- Why Might I Feel Helpless or Angry?

- Are Feelings of Depression Normal?

- What Should I Do If I Feel Discouraged, Frustrated, or Hopeless?

- How Can I Cope Better with My Emotions?

- Do I Need to Go to a Specialized Weight-Reduction Center to Lose Weight?

- Should I Seek Professional Counseling or Psychiatric Care?

- Am I Likely to Feel the Same Way About My Weight Throughout My Life?

In this chapter, we explore the relationship between emotions and obesity. We examine the ways people cope with their emotions and how those coping mechanisms might interact with weight gain or loss. We also discuss how underlying mental-health issues such as depression and anxiety can influence weight. The link between your emotions and your weight is significant, and learning how to understand what you are feeling and to address any possible issues will be a major part of any weight-loss strategy. Mental health and physical health are linked, and improving both can be an effective way to make positive changes in your life.

Is There a Normal Way to Feel About Having Excess Weight?

There are many emotions that you might experience because of having excess weight. You might feel sad, angry, frustrated, disgusted, anxious, or stressed. You might not be able to make any sense of your emotions, or you might have no idea how you are feeling at all. Maybe you have been dealing with underlying difficulties like depression or anxiety, and you feel that your problems have caused your weight gain. Or, you could have gained weight first and then began to experience negative emotions leading to depression, anxiety, or other issues (Scott et al, 2008).

In children and adolescents, excess weight can lead to low self-esteem, increased sadness, loneliness, or nervousness (Strauss, 2000). Children and adolescents also might have developed an underlying issue, like depression, and then became overweight. Some researchers have found that children and adolescents with *major depressive disorder* (MDD) might be at an increased risk for becoming overweight later in life (McElroy et al, 2004). Children and adolescents can experience a wide range of emotions about their excess weight.

The bottom line is that there is no "normal" way to feel about having excess weight. You can feel many different emotions depending on your own experience and nature. Recognizing how you are feeling, and when you started to feel that way, and then deciding where to go next are all important steps in improving your overall mental and physical health.

How Am I Likely to React When Others Tell Me That I Should Lose Weight?

Weight gain often provokes negative comments or criticism from others. These comments can come from family, friends, co-workers, classmates, bosses, children, or even doctors. Some people believe that weight is under the control of the individual and that weight gain is therefore the result of that person's own choices (Crandall et al, 2001). This can lead to more negative interactions by overweight or obese individuals with others. In dealing with these stigmatizing situations or comments, people react in a variety of ways (Myers &

Rosen, 1999; Puhl & Brownell, 2006), including heading off negative comments using positive self-talk; relying on faith, religion, or prayer; eating more food; and seeking social support from others.

These reactions are both positive and negative. How you tend to respond to these situations can affect your weight. Consider whether you have ever experienced a stigmatizing situation. Think about how you reacted. If those comments or situations caused you to become upset or stressed and your response to those emotions was to eat more, this could have caused you to gain more weight. It is never a good feeling when someone tells you that you need to lose weight, but learning to deal with these comments and the emotions they trigger in a healthy way is an important part of weight loss.

Why Might I Feel Helpless or Angry?

Helplessness and anger are normal emotions to experience if you are dealing with excess weight. There are several reasons why you might feel this way, including trying to achieve society's ideal body type, having underlying mental-health issues, experiencing *weight cycling* (more on this in a moment), or being stressed:

The Thin Ideal

One reason for these feelings, especially if you are female, might be that you have internalized society's "thin-ideal" body type (see Figure 2-1). TV, movies, advertisements, and other forms of media bombard society with images of thin women that can be difficult to ignore; they influence how you feel about your body (Thompson & Heinberg, 1999). Seeing and internalizing this ideal image of thinness but not being able to achieve it can surely be frustrating and lead to a negative *body image* or body dissatisfaction. Studies have shown that internalization of the thin-ideal is a key factor in body dissatisfaction in women (both in adults and adolescents) (Botta, 1999; Thompson & Stice, 2001; Yamamiya et al, 2005). Addressing this internalization, and understanding realistic and healthy body standards is a big step toward improving mental and physical health.

Underlying Mental-Health Issues

If you are currently struggling with depression, anxiety, or another underlying mental-health issue, this could be a contributing factor to your feelings of helplessness and anger. Treating these mental-health issues first is an important step to losing weight successfully and over the long term (McElroy et al, 2004). If you have not found the right help to get to the bottom of these mental-health issues first, you are likely to experience many negative emotions. Without first addressing your mental health, it could be a struggle to consistently keep weight off.

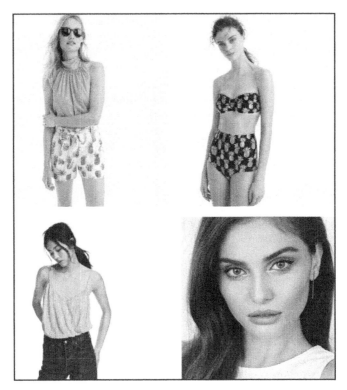

Figure 2-1: Clothing and make-up models depicting society's thin ideal.

Weight Cycling

Weight cycling, or, *yo-yo dieting*, is when you repeatedly engage in a pattern of losing weight for a period and then regain the weight back, or gain even more weight. Weight cycling could be associated with lower life satisfaction and disturbed eating, and possibly puts you at an increased risk for binge eating (Brownell & Rodin, 1994). These ups and downs might be making you feel helpless and angry, making it even more difficult to stay motivated on any weight-loss plan. Working to find the best sustainable weight-management plan, despite your highs and lows, can be a challenge. If weight cycling has been a serious issue for you, it could be helpful to work with a doctor or mental-health professional to modify your plan.

Stress

Stress is a contributing factor to weight gain and negative emotions for many individuals. Many people tend to respond to stress by eating more. In one study, adult women who reported stress also reported a greater drive to eat, including feelings of binge eating, hunger, and ineffective attempts to control their eating (Groesz et al, 2012). Other researchers have proposed that having a constant stressor in your life causes *cortisol* (a stress hormone) to be released in your body, which can cause you to crave more energy-dense (high-calorie) foods or cause you to gain and retain more fat in your abdominal area (Torres & Nowson, 2007). A recent study found that in adult men and women (54–87 years old), levels of cortisol (found in hair samples), were positively associated with persistence of obesity (the participants were obese when measured at multiple time points over a 4-year period). Obese individuals also had significantly higher cortisol concentrations in their hair samples than did the normal weight and overweight participants (Jackson et al, 2017). In another study, hair cortisol levels were also found to be increased in obese children (ages 8–12) when compared with a control group of normal-weight children (Veldhorst et al, 2014). It can be very frustrating to try to lose weight while your body is fighting against the weight loss due to chronic stressors. Think about your life and identify any consistent stressors. Is there anything you can do to decrease your stress?

Are Feelings of Depression Normal?

Before discussing the relationship between depression and weight gain, it is important for us to define depression. There are differences between feeling sad and being clinically depressed. Clinical depression (also known as the aforementioned MDD) is diagnosed when your sadness interferes with your everyday life. When your depressive symptoms get in the way of your work, school, social life, or other important areas, you might be experiencing depression. MDD is characterized by a variety of symptoms that can be recalled by the *mnemonic* (or memory tool) SIG: E CAPS. Each letter of the mnemonic stands for a different symptom.

- S: Sleep (increased or decreased)
- I: Interests (decreased)
- G: Guilt or preoccupation of thought
- E: Energy (decreased)
- C: Concentration ability (decreased)
- A: Appetite (either increased or decreased)
- P: Psychomotor (agitation or retardation [i.e., being too slowed down])
- S: Suicidal thoughts (American Psychiatric Association, 2013).

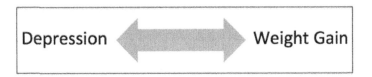

Figure 2-2: Depression and weight gain—a two-way street.

In addition, there must be depressed mood (most of the day, every day, or a marked decrease in interest or pleasure in almost all activities (i.e., *anhedonia*).

When these symptoms become so severe that they cause your work or school performance to suffer, you should seek help from a mental-health professional.

In thinking about the relationship between obesity and depression, it is helpful to think about it as a two-way relationship. You might have developed depression first and then gained weight, or you might have gained weight first and then developed depression (Figure 2-2).

In one study, researchers found that obese adults have a 55% increased risk of developing depression over time, and that depressed people have a 58% increased risk of becoming obese (Luppino et al, 2010). Another study found that adults who either were experiencing depression or had a life-time diagnosis of depression were each 60% more likely than those without depression to be obese (Strine et al, 2008). Children and adolescents with depression might also be at an increased risk for becoming overweight later in life (Goodman & Whitaker, 2002; McElroy et al, 2004).

It might be that due to depression, you lost interest in physical activity and this contributed to weight gain. Obesity might have contributed to other health problems or a physical disability, and your depression worsened (Dixon, Dixon, & O'Brien, 2003). If you were being treated for depression and were prescribed an antidepressant, the antidepressant might also have contributed to your weight gain. Certain antidepressants are more likely than others to cause weight gain (Fava, 1999).

There are many ways that depression and obesity interact. If you are experiencing depression or depressive symptoms along with weight gain, it is important to understand when the symptoms began in relation to your weight gain. In working to lose weight, it will be helpful to address any depressive symptoms with a professional to understand the root cause of your weight gain, especially if your depressive symptoms occurred first (McElroy et al, 2004).

What Should I Do If I Feel Discouraged, Frustrated, or Hopeless?

Seeking support can be helpful when you are feeling especially discouraged, frustrated, or hopeless. Whether you need encouragement, motivation, advice, or accountability, there are many resources available. The support you need might come from a family member or friend, a support group, a doctor, or from on-line sources. Think about how you are feeling, and which type of support might be best for you.

Face-to-face support groups like those offered by Weight Watchers provide encouragement, accountability, and motivation. Although Weight Watchers itself is an all-encompassing program that includes meal plans, those who attend face-to-face meetings tend to lose more weight (Mitchell et al, 2013). You can find other face-to-face support groups on-line, and they vary by city. Try searching through ObesityAction.org or Overeatersanonymous.org, to see if there are support groups in your area. Your doctor or mental-health professional might also have groups that meet weekly through their offices. Ask your doctor or therapist to help you find the right group for your specific needs.

On-line support groups offer a convenient way to receive the encouragement or advice you need while being able to remain relatively anonymous. In one study involving adults who visit the website SparkPeople.com, users enjoyed the convenience of the site, the ability to remain anonymous if they wanted, and the overall non-judgmental interactions on the site. Users' main activities on the site included giving or receiving personalized advice, encouragement, and motivation through shared stories of weight loss, seeking accountability or holding others accountable for their weight-loss goals, or participating in friendly competitions (Hwang et al, 2010). Hearing from others who have been on a similar journey can provide comfort, hope, and motivation in a time of hopelessness. If you do not feel comfortable participating in a face-to-face support group, the ease and anonymity of an on-line support group could be beneficial. Many programs, including Weight Watchers, offer on-line support in addition to in-person meetings. Search on-line for a forum or network that looks helpful to you, or ask your doctor or therapist to connect you with one.

If your support networks are not helping, and your emotions, weight, or other health issues are negatively affecting your everyday life, reach out to a doctor or other mental-health professional. Doctors who specialize in weight loss and weight-related issues can help you to navigate your options and determine the best resources for you.

How Can I Cope Better with My Emotions?

Learning to cope with your emotions in a healthy way will be a key component in managing your weight. Studies have found that obese adults have problems identifying and regulating their emotions (Kass et al, 2017). Not being able to identify and regulate emotions could lead to unhealthy eating behaviors and coping mechanisms and ultimately cause weight gain. Stress and negative emotions have been shown to make people eat (Groesz et al, 2012; Macht & Simons, 2000). Take a look at the statements in Table 2-1, a selection of items taken from the 52-item Eating and Appraisal Due to Emotions and Stress (EADES) questionnaire (Ozier et al, 2007), and think about how much you agree or disagree with each.

Table 2-1: Eating and Appraisal Due to Emotions and Stress

I use food to cope with my emotions
I eat when I am anxious
I am confident I can control my eating when I feel upset
I comfort myself with food
I eat when I am frustrated
I eat when I am sad
I eat when I am angry
I feel out of control when I eat
I eat when I am tired
It is difficult for me to stop eating when I am full
I overeat when I socialize
I eat when I am relieved
I am confident I can control my eating when I feel happy

Learning to pay attention to and understand your feelings, especially those feelings surrounding your eating habits, can help you to identify any problem areas and to develop healthy coping strategies. Understanding your feelings and habits is important not only for losing weight, but also for your overall mental health.

One strategy to improve emotional coping is *mindfulness*. Mindfulness involves learning to be present in the moment, to be aware of what you are experiencing, and to be aware of your bodily sensations in that moment. In brief, mindfulness means to pay attention (Germer, 2004). It is often defined as observing the immediate experience openly and without judgment (Bishop et al, 2004). There are different types of mindfulness-based therapies, and there have been many studies involving these different therapies as interventions for overweight and obese individuals. Mindfulness shows promise as a weight-loss intervention and could be a useful tool in learning to cope with your emotions in a healthy way.

One study about using mindfulness to decrease emotional eating invited half of participants (overweight and obese adult women) to take part in a mindful eating and stress-reduction program over the course of 9 weeks. Participants in this intervention group attended weekly 2.5-hour classes in addition to a final 7-hour retreat. The researchers found that participants in the intervention group were successful in increasing their mindfulness and responsiveness to bodily sensations, reducing their anxiety and eating response to external food cues, and reducing their emotional eating when compared with those in the control group. Additionally, those participants who reported the greatest improvements in mindfulness, responsiveness to bodily sensations, and chronic stress lost the most abdominal fat (Daubenmier et al, 2011).

In another mindfulness study, a group of adult participants took part in a Mindful Eating and Living (MEAL) intervention. The participants took MEAL classes for 6 weeks, with the goal of learning to understand hunger and satiety cues (clues to feeling full and satisfied) as well as emotional and cognitive states surrounding eating. All participants increased their mindfulness and cognitive restraint around eating, and decreased their weight, eating disinhibition, binge eating, and perceived stress (Dalen et al, 2010).

A third study involving adult women found that after attending 8 weekly sessions of a mindfulness-based intervention, participants showed significantly less body dissatisfaction as well as decreased emotional eating, external eating, and food cravings when compared with those in the control group (Alberts et al, 2012).

Speak to your doctor or mental-health professional about which type of mindfulness-based therapy might be right for you, especially if you believe that you need help sorting out your emotions as they relate to your eating habits.

Do I Need to Go to a Specialized Weight-Reduction Center to Lose Weight?

Yes, if it is recommended by your doctor or a professional counselor. If you are struggling with obesity and physical health problems, working with a weight-reduction center might be a useful option. Keep in mind that these treatment centers can vary in efficacy, and it is important to consider whether the weight-loss center is promoting a quick fix to lose weight or a cohesive plan that involves not only diet change, but also exercise, social support, and behavioral changes. Your doctor or mental-health professional should be able to guide you to effective weight-loss centers in your area.

Should I Seek Professional Counseling or Psychiatric Care?

Professional counseling or psychiatric care can be helpful for several reasons. If you are dealing with underlying depression, anxiety, or other mental-health issues, seeking professional help would be a positive step toward improving your health. If you experienced depression prior to your weight gain, addressing the depression with a professional counselor or psychiatrist first is an important step in successful weight loss (McElroy et al, 2004). If your depression or anxiety symptoms are severely interfering with your day-to-day life or if you are experiencing thoughts of suicide, you should seek help immediately.

If you believe that part of your weight gain stems from poor emotional regulation and you would like help learning how to cope with your emotions in a healthy way, reach out to a professional counselor or psychiatrist. A mental-health professional can provide you with the building blocks that you need to understand your emotions and help you to change your behavior to cope positively. They might also recommend specific group therapies or mindfulness interventions that can help you learn more about your emotions and your relationship with food.

If you think that you have an eating disorder, such as binge-eating disorder, you should seek professional counseling or psychiatric care. Individuals with binge-eating disorder generally eat large amounts of food in a short period and feel an overall lack of control during the episode. They might also eat large quantities of food when they are not actually hungry and feel embarrassed, disgusted, depressed, and guilty after the eating episodes (American Psychiatric Association, 2013).

Mental-health professionals can work with you to change any unhealthy behaviors and work through eating disorder symptoms. Mental health alone is not an answer to weight management, but it should be a part of any weight-loss plan, along with diet, exercise, and other doctor recommendations.

Am I Likely to Feel the Same Way About My Weight Throughout My Life?

You are likely to go through many ups and downs in your life, both emotionally and in regard to your weight. Your feelings will fluctuate. Learning to understand your feelings over time and to adjust when needed, to reduce stress, or change coping behaviors will help you to stay in control. By doing so, you will likely have more ups than downs. Understanding your emotions is just as important as is diet and exercise when it comes to managing your weight, and it is imperative that you are working on all of these areas to maintain a balanced life and a healthy weight.

Finding the right weight-management strategies for you and changing your lifestyle to implement those strategies successfully should lead to improvements in your overall physical and mental health. Addressing any underlying depression, anxiety, or other mental-health issues will also go a long way toward improving how you feel about yourself and your weight. Pay attention to your feelings, and do not be afraid to speak to others about what you are going through. If you need help sorting through your feelings, reach out to a friend, family member, doctor, or mental-health professional.

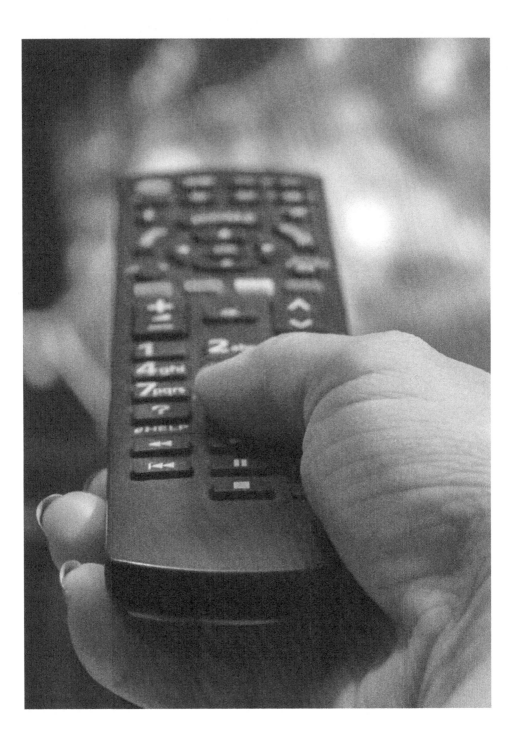

What Can I Learn From Portrayals Of Obesity In The Media?

Amy Vyas, MD

CHAPTER

In This Chapter

- What Can I Learn from Depictions of Obesity on Reality Television?

- What Stereotypes About Obesity Are Portrayed on Television and in Movies?

- Are There Any Complex Portrayals of Obese Characters on the Screen?

- Are There Any Dramatic or Comedic Television Series That Feature People Who Have Overweight and Obesity?

- What Should I Know About How Obesity Is Portrayed in Children's Shows and Movies?

- Should I Just Stay Away from My Television?

Introduction

Messages about obesity are conveyed both explicitly and implicitly on television and in film. These messages can be objectionable, validating, or confusing. Some are inaccurate and others are thought provoking. It is important to recognize that those messages conveying implicit or hidden attitudes might be the ones that society most takes for granted. Depictions of obesity on television might serve marketing aims or strive to be entertaining, and this purpose might proceed at the expense of accuracy, ethics, and social responsibility. Meanwhile, regardless of whether they are accurate, these representations have a very real impact on our choices and attitudes. Research has shown that the content of movies and television can affect the behaviors and health-related beliefs of viewers regarding alcohol use, tobacco use, and sexual behaviors (Throop et al, 2014). Carefully considering the impact of the content in televised media is essential for making responsible decisions regarding television and film consumption as it relates to obesity and health.

What Can I Learn from Depictions of Obesity on Reality Television?

As far as obesity goes, the term "reality television" is something of a misnomer. One of the original weight-loss reality shows, *The Biggest Loser*, saw contestants try to lose weight using a rigorous, often criticized as impractical or even dangerous, exercise and diet regimen for a prize of $250,000 dollars. The show was also criticized for insensitive images of contestants being weighed wearing minimal clothing and for portraying obesity of the contestants as fundamentally incompatible with a happy life. A follow-up show, *Losing It with Jillian*, saw former *Biggest Loser* trainer Jillian Michaels traveling the country to help people lose weight using a more holistic approach focused on lifestyle change. *The Biggest Loser* became something of a brand, leading to many other commercially successful products (e.g., cruises, books, weight-loss programs). However, another follow-up to *The Biggest Loser*, new in 2017, *The Big Fat Truth*, shows former contestants on *The Biggest Loser* who lost pounds on the show and then gained the weight (and more) back. Other successful reality show formats have included, *Extreme Makeover Weight Loss*, which follows contestants for more than a year, and *My Diet is Better than Yours*, which focuses on using diet planning to achieve weight loss.

Supersize vs Superskinny aired on television in the United Kingdom, and paired an overweight and underweight individual in a supervised environment in which they would live together and swap diets for 2 to 5 days. Their challenges were interspersed with documentary clips that provided education on health risks associated with being underweight or overweight, on healthy nutrition, and on weight-loss methods. Notably, the shows format included the individuals with underweight, overweight, and obesity reflecting on their respective eating habits, usually concluding that there was some component of emotionally-driven behavior (*emotional eating*) that had shaped their eating habits. The show treated both as potentially risky for health and well-being. Another British show, *Secret Eaters*, portrayed individuals who were either overweight or obese and underestimated or underreported their caloric intake. They completed food diaries and were followed by staff and private investigators, as if investigating a crime, observing their food intake (facts with which the individuals would later be confronted). The confrontation included photographic or filmed evidence of the secret eating behaviors, presented as if it were a crime; shame often followed. A dietitian would then provide advice for more healthful eating based on the data obtained by the private investigators.

You can glean some potentially useful ideas from reality television; however, the shows often provided misinformation, distortion, stigma, and commercial interests. You should remember that reality television generally functions by placing individuals into a contrived situation and seeks to entertain the audience; it does not rely on facts.

What Stereotypes About Obesity Are Portrayed on Television and in Movies?

Unfortunately, television did not start by featuring a series of rich and multi-dimensional characters who happen to have overweight and obesity. Studies have shown that overweight individuals are under-represented on television relative to their proportion in of the population, and when represented with obesity, characters are less likely to be cast as lead actors (Greenberg et al, 2003). Characters with overweight and obesity are more likely to serve as comic relief, are shown eating more frequently, but are less likely to be shown helping others, dating, or expressing physical affection. On the positive side, larger female characters were more likely to be respected, and larger male characters (relative to thin male counterparts) were less likely to be shown being ridiculed (Greenberg et al, 2003). The University of Connecticut Rudd Center for Food Policy and Obesity note that fictional TV characters with obesity are more often "portrayed as unattractive, lonely, or greedy" or shown "overeating unhealthy foods or being lazy (http://www.uconnruddcenter.org/weight-bias-stigma-media)."

Overall, the stereotypes of overweight and obese individuals are not positive. A common stereotype is the "fat, bumbling man, with the thin, capable, long-suffering wife" (Cohen, 2011) (as originated by Jackie Gleason in the 1950s show, *The Honeymooners*), and later continued in many forms, from *King of Queens* to the animated *The Simpsons* (one of the longest running shows in TV history), featuring the rotund, donut-scarfing nuclear power–plant worker Homer and his slender wife Marge. The "tragic fat girl" is lonely, overweight, awkward, bereft of the romance she so desperately desires, and often uses food to self-soothe. An example is the alternate "Fat Monica" version of Monica on the long-running hit sitcom *Friends*; this "what if" version of Monica is shown whining, missing out on romantic opportunities, and eating incessantly. Another version of this stereotype is played by Gwyneth Paltrow in the film *Shallow Hal*, about a superficial man who falls victim to a curse that causes him to see beyond shallow appearances to a person's true beauty. Confusingly, the Gwyneth Paltrow character is an obese woman with a wonderful personality, but is seen by the be-spelled Hal as slender and beautiful, so we are left to understand that her obesity either signifies unattractiveness or at the very least obscures her true beauty.

Becoming overweight or even gaining weight are seen as a character's demise. In the modern film classic, *Mean Girls*, one character takes revenge upon another by covertly feeding her weight-gain supplement bars, thus causing her to gain weight and lose the social status that apparently depended upon her slender physique. The various *Bridget Jones* movies show Bridget struggling with weight and voicing the expectation that these fluctuations will adversely affect her romantic prospects. Admittedly, Bridget's experience of having excess weight is handled less pejoratively than in the average film; after all, she is the main character and she does not need to lose weight to enjoy romantic success.

Another common stereotype is the "designated ugly fat friend," as featured as the protagonist in the film *The Duff*. This character is usually the sidekick, who is typically outshone by a main character in beauty and screen time (although she is often allowed a compellingly sassy or wise-cracking personality). Although *The Duff* would seem to subvert this trope, in the end the character is shown as desirable precisely because she learns to dress and to carry herself so that she does not appear overweight or ugly. Some of these mixed messages can communicate stigma in a manner that is ultimately more compelling because it is implicit.

Are There Any Complex Portrayals of Obese Characters on the Screen?

Not every depiction is burdened by stereotypes. *What's Eating Gilbert Grape?*, a 1993 motion picture directed by Lasse Hallstrom, starring Johnny Depp and Leonardo DiCaprio, followed a family living in a small Iowa town. The matriarch, Bonnie, played by Darlene Cates, had suffered the suicide of her husband and became housebound due to her struggles with obesity. Although she manages to extricate herself from her house to advocate for her disabled son, Bonnie is predominantly stuck at home. The actress herself had been housebound before being cast in the film and weighed as much as 548 pounds. The film thoughtfully approaches the difficulties her children face while balancing caring for their mother and coming of age, even though their mother is largely dependent upon them. The film examined the family dynamics around Bonnie's condition without passing judgment or implying fault.

The *Harry Potter* series is populated by a variety of characters with excess weight. Some characterizations are arguably burdened by stereotypes or unfavorable associations (such as the slovenly cousin Dudley, of whom it is implied that his obesity is related to his indulgent and lazy character, even though his "beefy" father is also overweight), whereas others seem designed to provide comic relief (e.g., the Fat Lady, who guards the dormitory). One of the sidekicks of Harry's evil nemesis is shown as an overweight dullard. However, the viewer is invited to accept other characters as having excess weight without a negative valence; not all the overweight characters are antagonists. The kindly Mrs. Dursley is described as "plump" in the books and the gentle, caring groundskeeper Hagrid is undeniably large. The complicated character, Professor Slughorn, is also overweight. Overall, the films present a wide variety of body types without associating an overweight body type with good or evil.

Are There Any Dramatic or Comedic Television Series That Feature People Who Have Overweight and Obesity?

The short-lived 2010 ABC network family series *Huge* followed teens and counselors at a weight-loss camp, but it was canceled after only 10 episodes. Kirstie Alley, of *Cheers* fame, had her own show, *Fat Actress*, which ran for one season on Showtime network; it depicted her struggles trying to get acting work while overweight. On the other hand, *Mike and Molly*, which was about a police officer and a teacher who meet at Overeaters Anonymous and fall in love, ran for six seasons. Though there were reports that *Mike and Molly* was canceled due to the female lead (Melissa McCarthy) losing weight, this was later debunked.

Before these, the hit show *Roseanne* ran on ABC for nine seasons mostly during the 1990s. Although not primarily concerned with issues relating to obesity, the show was considered groundbreaking at the time, not only for its focus on a working-class family, but also for having two lead characters who had excess weight without using weight as a comedic device or devolving into a stereotype. Although *Roseanne* was a sitcom, weight was handled with some realism; a later plot-line involved her husband suffering a heart attack. The show neither judged nor ignored the issue of weight.

What Should I Know About How Obesity Is Portrayed in Children's Shows and Movies?

Research has shown that children's health-related behaviors and attitudes can be shaped by the television shows and movies they consume (Throop et al, 2014). There is also a well-established relationship between hours spent watching television and the risk of becoming overweight (Gortmaker et al, 1996), which has been explained by the confluence of a complex array of factors, not only the sedentary aspect of television watching, but also the socio-demographics of increased television watching. Unfortunately, children and teens experience mixed messages from television and movies regarding obesity.

A study of 20 top-grossing PG- and G-rated movies from 2006 to 2010 showed that most contained "obesogenic" material (e.g., characters drinking sugary beverages or eating unhealthy snacks) as well as weight-related stigma (70% of the films stigmatized being overweight) (Throop et al, 2014). Children are often left to parse the complicated message of unhealthy weight-related behaviors being normalized while the same behaviors' potential effects are portrayed as undesirable.

The effects of stigma are extremely complicated. Total media exposure has been shown to have an association with stigmatizing attitudes in children toward other children who have obesity (Latner et al, 2007). Meanwhile, somewhat counterintuitively, exposure to stigma against people who are overweight is associated with increased caloric intake and also has an association with poor self-image, disordered eating, poor body image, and mood problems, even when controlling for *body mass index* (BMI), suggesting that experiencing the psychological ills of weight-related stigmatization do not depend on being overweight (Schvey et al, 2011).

Should I Just Stay Away from My Television?

A *Centers for Disease Control and Prevention* (CDC) panel was convened in 2006 to examine the troubled relationship between obesity and televised media consumption. After reviewing the evidence, they concluded that potentially feasible and meaningful interventions could include removing televisions from children's bedrooms, turning off televisions while eating, and providing physicians with resources that they could use to help patients reduce television consumption (Boulos et al, 2012). These interventions are simple but probably involve a significant amount of effort on the part of the individual.

The entertainment industry has a part to play, as well. Disney has promised to stop allowing advertisements featuring unhealthy snack foods on its cable channel (Throop et al, 2014). If such changes lead to meaningful shifts in obesity, corporate responsibility and ethical standards could follow, just as they have for other industries. The University of Connecticut Rudd Center for Food Policy and Obesity puts out guidelines for responsibly portraying individuals with obesity, including respecting diversity and avoiding stereotypes, using appropriate terminology (particularly using people-first language), providing balanced coverage, and using appropriate pictures that do not display pejorative or dehumanizing images (http://www.uconnruddcenter.org/resources/upload/docs/what/bias/media/MediaGuidelines_PortrayalObese.pdf).

It is probably not realistic to recommend ceasing to watch televised media, but just as with food, it is most prudent to make deliberate choices about what to consume. The HBO documentary series *The Weight of the Nation* offers a balanced, well-researched examination of obesity as a multi-faceted, dynamic problem. Remember that although documentaries are designed to present researched facts and accounts, comedy is meant to produce laughs, whereas reality television seeks to deliver entertaining but contrived scenarios; in addition, a great proportion of televised entertainment is a delivery vehicle for advertising. You should ask yourself, "How do I feel as I watch this?" and if the answer is "Diminished, depressed, or hopeless," this might be a sign that there is stigmatizing content. With a mindful approach to television and the cinema, there are opportunities for learning about how to face obesity in ourselves and in society.

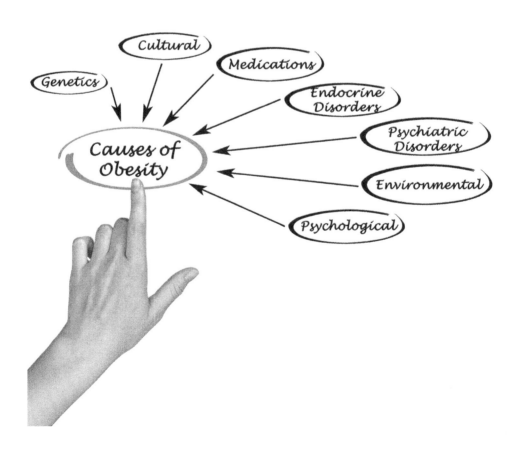

WHAT CAUSES OBESITY?

Karen J. Campoverde Reyes, MD

CHAPTER

In This Chapter

- Why Do People Gain Weight?
- Biological Factors
- Environmental Factors
- Genetic Factors
- Other Factors That Contribute to Obesity

Why Do People Gain Weight?

Given that the prevalence of obesity has been increasing at an alarming rate (in all age groups, and despite race, smoking, and education status) (Flegal, 2016), several theories about the causes of weight gain have been developed.

Set-Point Theory

The *set-point theory* is one of the most accepted and well-known theories of obesity. Many studies have shown that body weight is maintained in a stable range (the "set-point") during long periods despite the number of calories you consume (energy intake) and expend (amount of energy required for body functions). When someone decides to diet by decreasing the amount of food ingested, this creates energy restriction. When the body detects that there is a reduction in energy intake, it reduces its energy expenditures if the energy restriction persists. The body does its best to keep its usual weight. As soon as the energy–balance is restored and is detected to be adequate for the new (and lower) body weight, energy expenditure increases (Farias, 2011; Weinsier, 2001). The food you ingest, energy expenditure, and the way nutrients are stored in the body (e.g., fat and sugar deposits) determines your energy balance. To maintain a stable body weight, you should match your diet (fuel supply) with your body's energy requirements (Lopes, 2000). Your current environment also promotes excessive consumption of energy-dense foods, high in fat and sugar. These foods are usually affordable, accessible, and available in large portions. However, long-term exposure to these high-calorie diets might contribute to a set-point deviation and lead to a new steady-state weight range (Farias, 2011; Martinez, 2000; Wright, 2012).

The Predation-Release Hypothesis

The *predation-release hypothesis* suggests that random *gene* changes have occurred and favor genes that predispose to obesity. Each gene is like a recipe that gives our bodies specific instructions; each person owns a unique set of genes. However, identical twins share the same genetic code; this has allowed investigators to determine that there is a significant genetic contribution to metabolic efficiency and regulation of body weight. Some genes regulate *satiety* (the sensation of fullness), food intake, and regulate energy expenditure and *thermogenesis* (how much the body is able to burn at rest and with activity). Function of these genes might explain why some individuals have a *genetic susceptibility* to gain weight in the presence of a high-calorie diet or reduced daily physical activity (Martinez, 2000; Stanford, 2016).

Thrifty-Gene Hypothesis

According to the *thrifty-gene hypothesis*, evolution has favored weight retention; it protects our bodies against times of food scarcity and starvation. Our bodies have adapted more to protect us against weight loss than weight gain (Farias, 2011; Stanford, 2016).

Ethnic-Shift Hypothesis

The *ethnic-shift hypothesis* has shown that African-American women use energy more efficiently than do Caucasian women. When comparing metabolic differences among ethnic groups, studies suggest that African-Americans may regulate weight at a lower "set-point" and be at higher risk to regain lost weight (Farias, 2011; Weinsier, 2001; Martinez, 2000; Stanford, 2016).

Sedentary-Lifestyle Hypothesis

Weight gain is usually associated with a level of energy intake that is greater than energy expenditure. This energy intake relies on appetite regulation, which determines the quantity and quality of food eaten (Bayon, 2014). Low levels of physical activity decrease energy expenditure; as a result, sedentary behaviors contribute to weight gain. Current technological advances have made our lives easier. Even though these advances have made many of us more efficient, they have predisposed us to become more sedentary and consequently, to expend fewer calories. People who exercise more have a higher energy expenditure. This gives them a better capacity to regulate their energy intake while maintaining a lower weight than individuals who engage in lower levels of physical activity (Farias, 2011; Martinez, 2000; Stanford, 2016; Wright, 2012).

Drug-Induced Weight-Gain Hypothesis

Drugs, especially psychotropic medications (e.g., lithium, atypical antipsychotics), diabetic treatments, anti-hypertensives (e.g., beta-blockers such as metoprolol), steroid hormones, contraceptives, and antihistamines are associated with weight gain (Wright, 2012). For example, use of antipsychotics has been linked with significant weight gain within the first 10 weeks of use and is associated with increased appetite and an increased risk of obesity. Tricyclic antidepressants (TCAs) such as amitriptyline are also associated with a notable weight gain. Selective serotonin re-uptake inhibitors (SSRIs) such as paroxetine are used for depression and are also associated with weight gain. Anti-diabetic medications, including thiazolidinediones, sulfonylureas, glyburide, and insulin can induce significant weight gain. The weight gained from these medications might be small but the increasing prevalence of hypertension, diabetes, and depression could magnify their impact on increasing obesity rates (Dhurandhar, 2014)

Microbiome-Induced Obesity Hypothesis

Did you know that you have bacteria inside your body? Most of them are beneficial because they help to break down nutrients and synthetize vitamins. The adult intestine contains approximately 100 trillion microbes; this is called the *gut microbiota*, which is established at birth and is modified through infancy and later in life. Alterations in the microbiota early in life, such as exposure to candies or sweetened beverages at a very young age, can contribute to the development of obesity in adolescence and adulthood. Recently, microbial diversity in the gut (*Bacteroidetes* and *Firmicutes*) has gained the attention of the scientific community. Individuals with obesity seem to have reduced levels of *Bacteroidetes*, which coincides with studies done in obese mice. The diversity of bacteria in the gut regulates how the energy you obtained from food is used and how much fat is created in your body (Bäckhed, 2009). Studies are now trying to establish the role of the gut microbiota in the regulation of weight gain. Is it even possible that "poop pills" from a lean person could become the treatment for obesity? Investigators are trying to determine whether that could become one of the next steps in obesity management (Ducharme, 2016).

The Assortative-Mating Hypothesis

There is a genetic component to a high body-fat composition, and those with a genetic predisposition toward a higher *body mass index* (BMI) tend to reproduce at a higher rate. If those with stronger genetic predisposition for obesity reproduce at higher rates than do others, the population will become increasingly populated with individuals with obesity because the selection for genes that predispose to obesity will be favored (Stanford, 2016; Dhurandhar, 2014).

Fetal-Programming Hypothesis/Intrauterine Factors

The intrauterine environment influences the development of the growing fetus. Moreover, the offspring of nutrient-deprived mothers prefer high-fat diets and are more sedentary. Pre-pregnancy maternal obesity and excessive weight gain during pregnancy are both associated with increased birth weight and a higher rate of *macrosomia* in the offspring, which means that the newborn is significantly larger than average, with a weight greater than 8 pounds or 4,000 grams regardless of his or her gestational age. Children born to mothers before *bariatric* (weight-loss) *surgery* are more likely to have obesity than are children born to mothers after bariatric surgery. In addition, infants born either small or large for gestational age have an increased risk of obesity later in life, but minimizing gestational weight gain in pregnant women with obesity decreases their risk of having a large-for-gestational-age infant. All of this suggests that maternal over-nutrition or under-nutrition can influence outcomes of their offspring. Maternal weight gain during pregnancy might interact with genetic factors to render offspring more susceptible to developing obesity in young adult-hood (Dhurandhar, 2014; Reddon, 2016).

Biological Factors

What Are Calories and How Do They Affect My Weight?

Body weight is determined by energy intake and energy expenditures. When there is an imbalance between energy intake and expenditure, a change in body weight arises. If energy expenditure exceeds that of intake, a decrease in body weight will occur (Dokken, 2007). However, it is not a simple equation, because many factors both internal (e.g., genetic, hormonal, age-related changes) and external (e.g., stress, sleep quality, social anxiety, low income) affect body weight and regulation. (Source: Potential Contributors to Obesity Infographic [http://www.obesity.org/obesity/resources/facts-about-obesity/infographics/potential-contributors-to-obesity]).

Energy intake is measured in calories. A *calorie* is a unit of measurement of energy, and it is defined as the amount of heat necessary to raise the temperature of one gram of water one degree centigrade. Calories are essential because the body needs them for energy to support normal metabolic functions, growth and repair of tissues, and physical activity. Everyone requires a specific number of calories. A method to calculate one's caloric need is through the height in centimeters (H), weight in kilograms (W), age (A), sex, and physical activity of the individual by using the Harris-Benedict (HB) Equation for *resting energy expenditure* (REE):

Men REE = 66.5 + 13.8(W) + 5.0(H) − 6.8(A)
Women REE = 655.1 + 9.6(W) + 1.9(H) − 4.7(A)

Let's use the following example: You are a woman with a weight of 176 pounds, your height is 170 centimeters, and your age is 35. These values can be entered into the equation. But first, we need to transform pounds to kilograms. Because 1 kg is 2.2 pounds, you can divide 176 pounds by 2.2 and obtain 80 kg. Let's enter these values into the equation:

Woman REE = 655.1 + 9.6(80) + 1.9(170) − 4.7(35)
Woman REE = 655.1 + 768 + 323 − 164.5
Woman REE = 1,582 calories

This number of calories should suffice for someone who does light physical activities regularly (like walking slowly [i.e., while shopping, walking around the office], sitting at your computer, making the bed, eating, preparing food, and washing dishes).

If you get regular moderate-to-vigorous physical activity, your REE might need to be multiplied by a factor of 1.2 to 1.5, respectively, to account for extra calories that are needed during exercise. A factor of 1.2 represents an average amount of activity, whereas 1.5 would be a very high amount of activity. Let's assume that you are doing an average amount of activity. In this case, your caloric needs would be 1,582 calories × 1.2 = 1,898 calories per day. Some examples of moderate physical activities include sweeping the floor, walking briskly, slow dancing, vacuuming, washing windows, and shooting a basketball. On the other hand, some examples of vigorous physical activities include running (at least 5 mph), swimming, shoveling, playing soccer, jumping rope, carrying heavy loads (e.g., bricks). Although the HB equation is accurate for predicting the energy requirements within a healthy population, it is not as reliable for critically ill individuals. The REE represents the amount of energy expended by a person at rest.

Basal metabolic rate (BMR) is more precisely defined as the REE measured just after awakening in the morning. In practice, REE and BMR differ by less than 10%, so the terms can be used interchangeably. Even though the HB equation might be useful as a reference, it is important to keep in mind that muscles burn more calories at rest than does fat, so someone with low percentage of body fat and a high percentage of muscle will have a higher BMR than someone with the same weight but more fat and less muscle.

There are three major sources of energy in food, called *macronutrients*: carbohydrate, protein, and fat. Each of them provides a certain amount of energy: carbohydrates render 4 calories per gram, proteins give 4 calories per gram, and fat gives 9 calories per gram. Fats are much richer than other macronutrients; that is why you should watch for fat that you are ingesting. All together, they add up to the total daily calorie intake. Gaining or losing weight is not merely about counting calories; there are other factors besides calories that affect body expenditure to gain or lose weight (Prosch, 2013; Picolo, 2016; Roza, 1984; UCLA, 2005; Schakel, 2009)

What Are Fat Cells and How Do They Work?

Fat deposits in our bodies are housed in fat cells. We store fat around vital organs, such as the intestines and heart (to act as a soft padding), to act as a fuel reserve and to conserve body heat. The body makes fat cells, mostly from the fat and carbohydrates in our diet. An excess of fat cells can lead to insulin resistance, diabetes, and obesity-related metabolic abnormalities (Britannica, 2015; Tchoukalova, 2010). *Insulin resistance* is a term used to explain dysfunction in the normal metabolism of sugars and how they are stored. Women have higher percentages of fat when compared to men. Fat levels higher than in the normal range (18%–24% for men; 25%–31% for women) increase the risk of insulin resistance; this explains why people with diabetes are usually obese (Kahn, 2000).

Why Do Some People Carry More Excess Weight Than Others?

Why can Mary eat everything she wants and appear so slim? Why is John hungry all the time and never seems to reach satiety? Why does Edward need to run 3 miles every day to maintain his weight? Why do you seem to gain weight just by breathing? Some people carry more excess weight than others. This is the result of several factors that can affect the stability of their energy balance, as an excess of energy is often stored as body fat. Every creature on Earth has evolved through millions of years to use energy efficiently, which means to use less energy to perform specific tasks. We are designed to minimize the reduction in body weight during long periods of starvation to ensure our survival (Dokken, 2007; Dhurandhar, 2014). However, many things have changed through time that seem to facilitate obesity in some groups of people. There is little doubt that the process of modernization and economic re-structuring in both developing and developed countries has led to consequences that have affected nutritional and physical activity patterns. The rise in the prevalence of obesity in populations whose family weight history has been relatively constant provides proof that current environmental factors have an important role in its increase (Martinez, 2000). Let's explore each of the factors that can explain why some people carry more excess weight than do others.

Environmental Factors

Our current environment promotes over-eating and less physical activity. Only half of adults 18 years and older meet the 2008 federal physical activities guidelines for participation in leisure-time aerobic and muscle-strengthening activities (CDC, 2014). Roughly one-fourth of youth aged 12 to 15 years old are engaged in moderate-to-vigorous physical activity, including activities both within and outside of school, for at least 60 minutes each day (Fakhouri, 2014). Many cities have disproportionally grown and are no longer designed for their inhabitants to walk or to use their bikes to move freely from one place to another. If you live in a city with sidewalks and biking trails, you can consider yourself lucky.

Although most people would agree that technology has made our lives easier, it promotes sedentary behaviors. More than half of the world's population now has internet access and two-thirds of the global population now use mobile phones. Nearly 2.8 billion people around the world currently use social media at least once per month, with more than 91% of them doing so via mobile devices (Digital in 2017: Global overview,

2017). Access to the internet, videogames, series and movies on-line has also had a health impact on many populations by reducing our calorie expenditure. You can even get food through internet applications, which facilitate purchases of generous high-calorie portions. But environmental influences do not stop there; fast-food restaurants, convenience stores, vending machines at schools and offices—all of these have an adverse impact on your weight. Besides this, today's accelerated lifestyle encourages the consumption of highly processed foods, which are generally high in sugar, fat, and sodium. All of these products are heavily advertised through media, aiming at adults and children. Both pre-packaged and non-perishable, many of them seem convenient, practical, and even financially friendly. However, a diet that is low in fruits and vegetables along with a high intake of meat and highly processed foods has been associated with *visceral adiposity*, which refers to fat that is stored around vital organs (such as the liver, pancreas, and kidneys) (Wright, 2012; Dokken, 2007; Dhurandhar, 2014; Burgermaster, 2017).

What about the consumption of *sugar-sweetened beverages* (SSBs)? Their consumption will be more likely to cause an increase in body fat mass in any healthy lean adult and weight gain among obese adults. The *American Heart Association* (AHA) recommends that added sugars not exceed 100 to 150 kcal/day and has identified SSBs as the primary source of added sugars and calories, with no true nutrients, in our current diets.

How about drinking *artificial sweetened beverages* (ASBs)? Even though they are marketed as "healthy alternatives" due to their lack of calories, they stimulate sweet taste receptors, which could increase appetite, induce a preference for sweet-tasting foods, and result in over-consumption of solid foods due to awareness of the low-calorie content of ASBs. Systematic reviews of observational studies indicate that intake of ASBs is linked with increased BMI in both children and adults. Absence of evidence to support the role of ASBs in the prevention of weight gain and the lack of studies on other long-term effects on health strengthen the position that ASBs should not be promoted as part of a healthy diet. More recently, published data suggests that artificial sweeteners might contribute to the development of *glucose intolerance* by altering the composition and functions of gut microbiota (Burgermaster, 2017; Borges, 2017). Even though water is the healthiest option, breaking habits is a challenge for many; drinking water is the best long-term decision when trying to manage weight. However, it is imperative to keep in mind that weight gain is multi-factorial, and cutting out sweetened beverages is only one step toward a healthier life.

Anthropological studies also have shown that food choices of employees are influenced by the worksite. This is not limited to the meals that are available in the cafeterias, but also takes into account the support and help employees receive from their co-workers in meeting individual health and nutrition goals. In general, having healthier foods in the work environment is well accepted and appreciated. However, because work fatigue and overtime work also have been associated with weight gain, many aspects of the work environment should be re-assessed to avoid them (Devine, 2007).

Socioeconomic background influences the quality of the food we buy. Which one is more affordable: a pizza or a salad? It has been shown that living in lower income neighborhoods is associated with a lower-quality diet; moreover, there are large racial disparities in healthy food availability that could lead to a low-quality diet and to obesity (Franco, 2009). New Yorkers with a lower socioeconomic status and from minority sub-groups consume more SSBs and have higher BMIs (Burgermaster, 2017).

In addition, there is a *thermal neutral zone* (i.e., the range where the standard healthy adult can maintain normal body temperature without needing to use energy above and beyond normal basal metabolic rate [25°C–30°C; 77°F–86°F]). Metabolic rate increases by 7% to 17% for every one-degree Celsius rise in core body temperature; this rate increases with heat exposure. Further, a higher core temperature decreases food intake and results in food choices with a lower energy density. With the prevalence of air conditioning we have reduced our exposure to this range; evidence suggests that being outside the thermal neutral zone might influence our energy balance. However, further studies are required to demonstrate that chronic heat exposure changes energy balance enough to influence our body weight (Dhurandhar, 2014). It is certainly unappealing to embrace the idea of life without the comfort of air conditioners.

Genetic Factors

But, you still might be thinking, why do some people struggle so much with their weight if they seem to eat healthy and try to be active? Always keep in mind that obesity is the result of multiple factors. However, there are indeed some people whose genetic lottery plays against them and predisposes them to gain weight easier than other people. The role of inheritance has long been recognized to affect intake and expenditure of the energy balance, given that some genes are involved in food intake control, the regulation of thermogenesis, and energy expenditure; these genes might specifically be affected by dietary intake and composition, which might explain why some people easily gain weight whenever they decide to "sin" and eat a slice of pizza (high in fat and carbohydrates). Individuals genetically predisposed to obesity appear to be less efficient at oxidizing fat intake, and when the consumption of carbohydrate is high, there is an increase in the formation of new fat cells in the body, which is known as *de novo lipogenesis*. These genetic predisposition mutations can be classified into two groups: *monogenic mutations* and *polygenic mutations* (Martinez, 2000).

Monogenic obesity comes from a single gene mutation and can be divided into syndromic or non-syndromic. *Syndromic obesity* refers to obesity that occurs with a distinct set of observable features (*phenotypes*) that result from genetic inheritance (*genotype*). *Intellectual disability* (formerly called mental retardation), *dysmorphic features*, and organ-specific developmental abnormalities are part of the clinical picture, along with obesity in this type of mutations. Non-syndromic forms are caused by mutations or structural variations in genes involved in the decrease of the hormone that suppresses appetite (*leptin*) and are mainly characterized by obesity caused by excessive hunger, called *hyperphagic obesity*. The people who are carriers of these mutations are extremely rare and lead to an early-onset extreme obesity (Dokken, 2007; Reddon, 2016).

Polygenic mutations imply that there are DNA variations in several genes, each with relatively small effect. Hundreds of these variants with small-to-modest effect plus other factors such as the socioeconomic environment and lifestyle, diet, sex and age, as well as alcohol consumption might contribute to the development of obesity (Reddon, 2016).

Socioeconomic environment and lifestyle

The proportion of variability in BMI attributable to *genetic variation* is increased among people born after the establishment of a modern *"obesogenic"* environment. Socioeconomic research indicates that higher educational status is associated with a decreased risk of obesity, but it has been suggested that BMI in adolescence is positively correlated with the level of education of the parents. *Twin studies* have shown that a high level of physical activity can substantially reduce the influence of genetic factors on BMI in both young and older adults. Therefore, *genetic predisposition* to obesity can be blunted in part through physical activity. Lifestyle factors and socioeconomic background can significantly modify the impact of obesity-predisposing gene variants (Reddon, 2016; Wardle, 2008).

Diet

Studies in Mediterranean, Asian, Caucasian, Hispanic, and Caribbean populations, suggest that a high daily energy intake, high-fat intake, or high saturated-fat intake (e.g., high intake of fried foods) can amplify the effect of certain genes that predispose to obesity risk in children, adolescents, and adults. Increased intake of SSBs has also been shown to increase the impact of obesity genes. Fat mass and obesity–associated gene (*FTO* gene) and its variants, *Apolipoprotein* A (APOA2 and APOA5), *single nucleotide polymorphisms* (SNPs), are all genetic mutations that have shown the strongest associations with obesity predisposition when combined with diet (Reddon, 2016; Livingstone, 2016; Voisin, 2015).

Sex and age

Sex-specific genetic effects on BMI have been observed in adolescents as well as in adults. Females are generally more likely to develop morbid obesity than males, which suggests that there might be some differences between men and women in the genetic factors that influence variation in BMI. Heritability of obesity also varies with age (BMI changes from adolescence to young adulthood, and from young adulthood to adulthood); obesity is a heritable trait. Mobility usually decreases with age, contributing to obesity, too (Reddon, 2016, Schousboe, 2003).

Alcohol consumption

Many people enjoy an occasional beer or glass of wine. But what is the impact of alcohol on your weight? Alcohol energy (7 kcal/g) can be a contributing factor to weight gain. If someone consumes a light-to-moderate amount of alcohol, there is no obesity risk. Heavy drinking and binge drinking do have an association with excess body weight. It has been found that one month of daily beer consumption (equivalent to 12g/day of alcohol for women and 24 g/day for men) does not result in significant increases in BMI compared to those who abstain. *Biceps skin fold* was the only *anthropometric measurement* that was increased in the participants who had beer. However, alcohol can influence BMI if there is the genetic predisposition. For example, the consumption of alcohol in Asian people increased the effect of SNPs in BMI. This pattern has also been shown with other mutations in African Americans (Reddon, 2016; Gregory Traversy, 2015).

Other Factors That Contribute to Obesity

Psychological Factors

There are psychological and behavioral risk factors that predispose people to obesity. In those with depression, for each additional depressive symptom reported, the possibility of obesity onset increases four times. Depressed individuals eat to provide comfort or distraction from negative emotions (*"comfort food"*) in an attempt to raise serotonin levels—the "happy neurotransmitter"—in the brain; thus, they consume excessive amounts of carbohydrate-rich foods in an effort to regulate serotonin levels. Also, weight-control behaviors can increase the risk for binge eating, which in turn results in weight gain (Stice, Presnell, Shaw, & Rohde, 2005).

Maternal Age

Through the past decades, childbearing has been occurring later in life. The mean age at first birth has steeply increased from 21.4 in 1970 to 26.4 years in 2015 (Martin, 2017). These changes in maternal age at the time of delivery might have affected the susceptibility of offspring to increased adiposity and obesity. Evidence suggests that positive shifts in the maternal age distribution might influence the developing fetus and the likelihood of obesity in those offspring. Older mothers are more likely to develop co-morbidities and metabolic abnormalities during pregnancy, which can influence obesity, insulin resistance, and *hypertension* in their offspring (Dhurandhar, 2014).

Smoking Cessation

Smoking has been associated with a lower BMI and its cessation is associated with weight gain. The mechanisms through which this happens are not clear, but it is well known that *nicotine* (one of the main components in cigarettes) is a *thermogenic agent* and that smoking decreases appetite (Dhurandhar, 2014).

Sleep Debt

Do you sleep enough? Sleep is a restorative process that plays an important role in the balance of psychological, emotional, and physical health. Increasing evidence suggests that not obtaining enough sleep might be associated with adverse health effects such as obesity. Sleep debt tends to increase food intake, energy storage, and the likelihood of diabetes and heart disease. People who are sleep deprived tend to have increased evening concentrations of the stress hormone *cortisol*, which has been shown to suppress appetite and increase hunger by causing the decrease of leptin (the substance that suppresses appetite) and the increase of *ghrelin* (the hormone that stimulates appetite). Despite physical activity, weight gain due to sleep debt affects children, adolescents, and adults. Some studies also have shown that people who sleep less than 7 hours per night have higher BMIs and are more likely to be obese when compared to people who sleep at least 7 hours (Bayon, 2014; Karine, 2004; Gangwisch, 2005; Dhurandhar, 2014).

Summary

In this chapter, we pointed out the main factors that lead to obesity. Obesity depends on multiple factors that go far beyond caloric intake and expenditure. Evidence suggests the existence of genes that predispose to weight gain. Also, there are race, gender, age, psychological, and socioeconomic factors that influence this outcome. Healthy habits, such as regular physical activity, consistent sleep patterns, and a balanced diet that meets metabolic requirements, can counteract those influences that are beyond your control. The human body's nature is to keep weight in a certain range, and as a matter of survival, it is still adapted to protect individuals against weight loss compared to weight gain. Just like the little genetic mutations that add together to create a modest effect in weight gain, the commitment to small changes of unhealthy habits can sum up to a huge impact toward an improved and longer life.

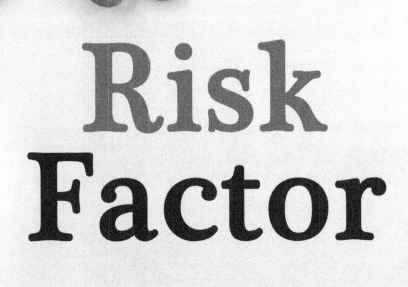

HOW CAN I TELL WHETHER I AM AT RISK FOR DEVELOPING OBESITY?

Ethan Lazarus, MD

CHAPTER

In This Chapter

- What Is the Goal of Obesity Screening?
- What Makes a Good Screening Test?
- How Can Factors That Contribute to Obesity Be Categorized?

What Is the Goal of Obesity Screening?

Like any disease, obesity is associated with a variety of health consequences ranging from risk for other diseases (like *diabetes* and *high blood pressure*) to decreased quality of life. In severe cases, obesity can also shorten your life span. For this reason, it is important to identify who does and who does not have obesity as well as to find out who might be *at risk* to develop obesity.

By identifying those at risk, we can take steps to prevent further weight gain and prevent obesity. And, if we catch obesity early, we can intervene before it becomes severe. Without screening, many individuals won't know whether their weight poses a risk to their health.

We can even screen children for obesity risk. It has long been observed that 40% of overweight children continue to be heavy during adolescence, and 75% to 80% of adolescents with obesity will remain obese as adults (https://www.ncbi.nlm.nih.gov/pmc/articles/PMC3005642/).

What Makes a Good Screening Test?

Body Mass Index

The most common tool used to screen for obesity is called the *body mass index* (BMI). However, many now agree that it is not the best tool. BMI is a good screening tool because it is free, easy to reproduce, and without risk.

The history of the BMI is quite interesting. It was invented in 1832 by Adolphe Quetelet, a Belgian mathematician and astronomer. He observed that, other than shortly after birth and during puberty, "weight increases as the square of the height (https://www.ncbi.nlm.nih.gov/pubmed/17890752)." The term, "body mass index," was coined by Ancel Keys in 1972 (https://en.wikipedia.org/wiki/Body_mass_index).

BMI is calculated by taking your weight in kilograms and dividing it by your height squared. Or, if you prefer Imperial units, take your weight in pounds, and divide it by your height squared, and then multiply by 703, like this:

$$\frac{\text{Weight (pounds)}}{(\text{weight in inches} \times \text{height in inches})} \times 703 = \text{BMI}$$

For example, if you are 200 pounds and 5 feet 10 inches tall (70 inches), your BMI would be:

$$\frac{200}{(70 \times 70)} \times 703 = 28.7 \text{ kg/m}^2$$

According to the World Health Organization (WHO), a BMI that is too low can indicate malnutrition, an eating disorder, or another health problem, whereas a BMI that is too high can indicate obesity. These ranges of BMI are valid only as statistical categories (see Table 5-1).

Table 5-1: Correlating BMI Scores

BMI (kg/m²)	Category
Less than 18.5	Underweight
18.5–24.9	Normal (healthy weight)
25–29.9	Overweight
30–34.9	Class 1 obesity – mild obesity
35–39.9	Class 2 obesity – moderate obesity
40 or greater	Class 3 obesity – severe obesity

Although the ranges listed in Table 5-1 are observed for classification purposes in the United States, other countries use different definitions. Some ethnicities have a high health risk even at BMI measurements considered "normal" in America. For example, practitioners in both Hong Kong and Japan consider a BMI greater than or equal to 25 to be obese.

Also keep in mind that these are adult ranges—for children aged 2 to 20 years, you can still calculate a BMI; however, instead of using fixed cut-offs like those in Table 5-1, it is better to plot them on a BMI-for-age graph and to calculate their BMI percentile, like we monitor childrens' height and weight. Children with a BMI between the 85th and 95th percentile are overweight, and above the 95th percentile (meaning that they are heavier than 95% of all children) have obesity.

Body Composition

Although BMI is useful for estimating health risk, another way to think about your weight is *body composition*; that is, "How much of your body is fat weight versus lean weight?" Body composition is not typically used as a screening tool because there are lots of ways to measure it and the results achieved by the different techniques are not always the same. It requires specialized equipment, so it is more difficult to obtain than is BMI. Moreover, some of the technologies available might not be suitable for all people (for example, body-fat scales use an electrical current and are not considered safe for people who are pregnant or who have a pacemaker).

Nevertheless, body composition is useful to estimate your level of fitness. Your body is made up of fat, bone, water, and muscle. Body composition measurements can provide you with an estimate of the amount of your body that is fat. Two people at the same BMI can have a very different body compositions—for example, one might have a sedentary life style and have low muscle weight and high fat weight—and therefore have a high health risk, whereas another might be very active and physically fit, having a high muscle weight and low fat weight—and therefore have a low health risk.

Many techniques are used to measure body composition. The most common is called *bioelectrical impedance analysis* (BIA). BIA is used on the different body composition devices incorporated into scales and/or hand-held units. BIA uses the resistance of electrical flow through the body to estimate body fat. It can be affected by hydration status, although some scales are more resistant to this effect than are others. BIA devices range from inexpensive household scales to very expensive medical-grade scales.

The most accurate and increasingly available technology is *dual energy X-ray absorptiometry* (DEXA or DXA) *scanning*. Many people are familiar with this technology because it is used for *osteoporosis* screening. The measurements are highly reproducible making them excellent for research purposes.

For decades, the "gold standard" way to measure body composition was underwater weighing. The individual is placed in a pool of water and fully submersed. By doing this, we can measure the person's volume, and then calculate their body composition. When done properly, underwater weighing is very accurate.

Like underwater weighing, *air displacement plethysmography* measures air displacement instead of water displacement. This way you don't need to get wet! For this test, you sit in an instrument that looks like a large egg and the machine determines how much air you displace.

Another tool calculates skin-fold measurements, using *calipers*. Many different areas can be measured, and there are formulas to convert skin-fold thicknesses to body fat percentages. However, there can be a lot of variability from person to person, and it requires special training for the individual to be able to calculate skin-fold measurements properly.

After you know your body-fat percentage, you can calculate your fat weight and your lean weight, also called the *fat-free mass*. Thus, if your body-fat percentage is 25% and you weigh 150 pounds, your fat weight is .25 × 150 = 37.5 pounds, and your lean weight (or fat-free mass) is the difference, or 112.5 pounds. So, if you are going on a weight-loss program and lose 25 pounds, and your follow-up body-fat percentage is 20%, you now have .20 × 125 = 25 pounds of fat, and 100 pounds of lean.

There is not one agreed-upon definition for ideal body-fat percentages, but there is a good review of this by the *American College of Sports Medicine* (http://www.livestrong.com/article/426250-acsm-body-fat-guidelines/). Also, your body-fat percentage usually increases as you age. Therefore, we don't expect you to have the same body-fat percentage when you turn 70 years old that you had when you were 20. Tables 5-2 and 5-3 show some sample body-fat percent ranges at different ages for men and women.

Table 5-2: Body-Fat Percentages for Men

	Age in Years				
	20–29	30–39	40–49	50–59	60+
Highly athletic	7.1–11.7	11.3–15.8	13.6–18	15.3–19.7	15.3–20.7
Above average fitness	11.8–15.8	15.9–18.9	18.1–21	19.8–22.6	20.8–23.4
Average fitness	15.9–19.4	19–22.2	21.1–24	22.7–25.6	23.5–26.6
Below average fitness	19.5–25.8	22.3–27.2	24.1–28.8	25.7–30.2	26.7–31.1
Well below average fitness	≥25.9	≥27.3	≥28.9	≥30.3	≥31.2

Table 5-3: Body-Fat Percentages for Women

	Age in Years				
	20–29	30–39	40–49	50–59	60+
Highly athletic	14.5–18.9	15.5–19.9	18.5–23.4	21.6–26.5	21.1–27.4
Above average fitness	19–22	20–23	23.5–26.3	26.6–30	27.5–30.8
Average fitness	22.1–25.3	23.1–26.9	26.4–30	30.1–33.4	30.9–34.2
Below average fitness	25.4–32	27–32.7	30.1–34.9	33.5–37.8	34.3–39.2
Well below average fitness	≥32.1	≥32.8	≥35	≥37.9	≥39.3

Other Measurements

We can also estimate your health risk from your weight by doing measurements around your waist, your hips, and your neck.

Waist Circumference

To measure your waist circumference, you should wrap a tape measure around your body (above your hip bone and below your rib cage). A measurement of 35 inches or greater is considered unhealthy for women. For men, a measurement of 40 inches or more is considered unhealthy.

Waist-to-Hip Ratio

To measure around your hips, wrap a tape measure at the widest part of your buttocks or hip. Then, calculate your waist-to-hip ratio (WHR) by dividing your waist measurement by your hip measurement. For women, a ratio of more than 0.8 is considered at higher risk, and for men, it is more than 1.0, because there is more abdominal fat.

Neck Circumference

To calculate your neck circumference, simply wrap a tape measure around your neck (not too tight! Be sure that you can breathe comfortably!) A measurement of 16 inches or more in women, or 17 inches or more in men is a risk factor for *sleep apnea*. Sleep apnea is a condition in which the airway can close intermittently at night resulting in poor oxygen flow to the brain. It is a risk factor, and a contributor to obesity. If you have an elevated neck circumference and/or symptoms of sleep apnea (like morning fatigue, morning headache, snoring, or excessive daytime sleepiness), be sure to talk to your doctor about screening for sleep apnea.

How Can Factors That Contribute to Obesity Be Categorized?

Contributors to Developing Obesity

People gain weight for a wide variety of reasons (medical, psychological, physical, and functional).

It's far more complicated than the age-old "calories in/calories out" mantra would suggest. In fact, we know that most of the risk for developing obesity is *genetic*. We know that if a child has a parent with overweight, they have a 40% increased risk for becoming overweight themselves. If both parents have overweight or obesity, this risk is 80%. (https://www.ncbi.nlm.nih.gov/pmc/articles/PMC3005642/) Although there are some single-gene mutations that can cause severe obesity, for most of us, there are hundreds if not thousands of different *genes* involved in body-weight regulation. Given the proper environment, some people are very likely to develop obesity, whereas others aren't. Have you ever noticed that some people can eat whatever they want and not gain weight, whereas others, despite carefully monitoring everything they eat, become quite heavy?

If we think about genetics "loading the gun" to develop obesity, the environment "pulls the trigger." A person with a high genetic risk for developing obesity can be at higher risk if they live in a big city where they have a high-stress job that requires sitting most of the day, and struggle to make ends meet (as opposed to. . .if they won the lottery, lived in a tropical paradise, and became a yoga instructor).

Our American environment makes maintaining a normal body weight increasingly difficult. Our food supply is abundant, and we are exposed to an ever-increasing array of delicious but unhealthy foods. We are eating more sugar than ever. The average American is estimated to consume between 150 and 170 pounds of refined sugar every year! 100 years ago, the average consumption was just 4 pounds per year. We rely on cars and public transportation to get around; and since the advent of the personal computer and with the widespread use of the internet, we have become largely sedentary at work.

Medical Contributors to Obesity

Medical contributors to obesity include other diseases, like diabetes and sleep apnea. These diseases can directly cause obesity. Conversely, obesity can directly cause these diseases. Typically, as one condition becomes worse, so does the other. Fortunately, with weight loss, many of these diseases can improve, too. In fact, studies have shown that losing 6% of your body weight can reduce your risk of developing type 2 diabetes by roughly 60%. In addition to other diseases that directly cause weight gain, many prescription medications can also induce weight gain. These drugs include those used for diabetes, high blood pressure, contraception, depression and bipolar disorders, inflammation, seizures, and even insomnia.

Obesity has also been associated with many types of cancer, including cancer of the breast, ovary, uterus, stomach, pancreas, gallbladder, and even prostate.

Psychological Contributors to Obesity

Psychological contributors to obesity include diseases like depression and binge-eating disorder. We all eat for "emotional" reasons. We eat because it helps us feel better. We eat because we are stressed, anxious, happy, or fatigued. We eat in front of the television and consume more food than when we are focused on a task—or the so called "mindless eating." We skip meals all day at work and then can't stop eating at night. Or, we eat as part of our job when meeting with clients. Whatever the reason, food plays an important role in our personal lives and in our psychological health.

Physical and Functional Contributors to Obesity

Physical and functional contributors to obesity include things like joint pain and fatigue. These types of conditions can make it difficult to exercise or difficult just to get around. They affect our ability to do the things we'd like to do and decrease our quality of life. In fact, a recent study found that more than 200 diseases are related to obesity (Yuen M, et al, 2016).

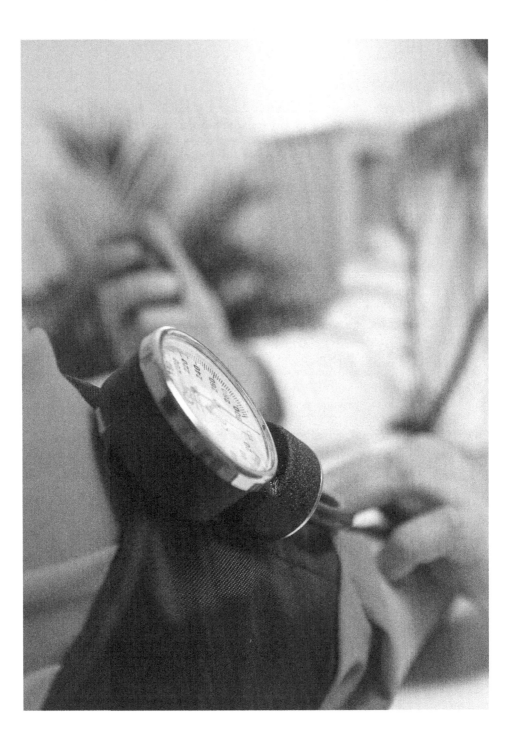

WHAT ARE THE MEDICAL COMPLICATIONS OF OBESITY?

Rajavi Shah, MD; Carl Palad, BS; and Ajay Shah, MD

CHAPTER

How Can Obesity Lead to Medical Complications?

The obesity epidemic is one of the biggest health threats in the United States; as a result, it has garnered significant attention from physicians, politicians, and the public. The symptoms of *overweight* and *obesity* involve not only physical manifestations, but they also affect one's behavior and psychological self. These additional components increase the complexity of the disease and its solutions. Unfortunately, rates of overweight and obesity in children and adults continue to climb despite recent interventions that involve increased community and governmental efforts in the prevention and management of these conditions (Obesity Rates & Trends, 2017; Strategies to Prevent Obesity, 2017). A serious concern linked with overweight and obesity is the wide range of associated medical complications. Thus, solutions for the management of overweight and obesity must consider a range of complications (e.g., *hypertension, type 2 diabetes mellitus*). This chapter aims to improve your knowledge of various medical complications associated with overweight and obesity.

Frequently, concern about developing a medical complication associated with obesity motivates behavioral change. As is true with many things regarding our health, knowledge is power; therefore, the idea behind this chapter is to educate you and your family about potential medical complications that are associated with obesity. As you read this chapter, don't let it scare you! The more you know, the more you'll be able to motivate yourself and your loved ones to make changes.

There are many causes of obesity; however, this chapter focuses on the complications of obesity itself. Our goal is to cover some of the common and significant obesity-related complications, in an easy-to-follow format.

Which Cardiovascular Conditions Are Worsened by Obesity?

Hypertension

Hypertension (*high blood pressure*) is a major consequence of overweight and obesity. Approximately one-third of Americans have hypertension, and in nearly one-third (30%) of them, that statistic can be directly attributed to overweight or obesity (Hypertension in the United States, 2015). Before discussing how high blood pressure is affected by obesity, let us first define the condition. In our *circulatory system*, blood travels through tube-like vessels (*arteries*) to deliver the oxygen and nutrients that our organs need. *Blood pressure* is the amount of force used to move blood through the walls of those arteries. The pressure originates from the rhythmic pumping of blood by the heart to the arteries. Because the heart is a muscle, it contracts and relaxes, producing two kinds of blood pressure: *systolic* and *diastolic*. When the heart contracts, it pumps blood into the arteries. The pressure in those arterial walls during contraction is the systolic pressure. When the heart relaxes, it receives blood from the body. This pressure, during relaxation, is the diastolic pressure, which is lower than the systolic pressure. Blood pressure is read as two values: systolic over diastolic blood pressure (Chronic Hypertension, 2017).

Table 6-1 displays the guidelines used by health-care providers to determine normal versus high blood pressure. High blood pressure (hypertension) is defined as the increase in resistance for the heart to pump blood through the walls of narrowing vessels. An increase in blood pressure can be caused by a variety of *genetic* and environmental factors. A study by Dua and colleagues (2014) found a link between high blood pressure and *body mass index* (BMI), which is the ratio of weight to height. BMI ratings between 25.0 and 29.9 are considered overweight, whereas having a BMI greater than or equal to 30.0 qualifies for obesity. High BMI values contribute to increased blood pressure readings. Additionally, high blood pressure can develop due to the increased workload that arteries must manage to deliver oxygen and nutrients to the excess fat tissue present in those who are overweight or obese (high BMI). Diets high in *cholesterol* and sodium can lead to the production of *arterial plaques*, which block blood flow in arteries and increase the blood pressure (Chronic Hypertension, 2017; Dua et al, 2014). Another explanation of how hypertension is caused by obesity involves the relationship between the elevated heart rates observed in patients with overweight and obesity. Raising the heart rate (the number of heart beats per minute) can make it more difficult for blood to travel through the arteries, leading to hypertension (Chronic Hypertension, 2017). Hypertension, linked to overweight and obesity, can give rise to further complications, such as heart disease and type 2 diabetes mellitus.

Table 6-1: Guidelines for Blood Pressure Readings in Adults (Basile and Bloch, 2016)

Blood Pressure Category	Systolic (mm Hg) (Upper Number)		Diastolic (mm Hg) (Lower Number)
Normal	Less than 120	and	Less than 80
Elevated	120–129	and	Less than 80
High Blood Pressure (Hypertension) Stage 1	130–139	or	80–89
High Blood Pressure (Hypertension) Stage 2	140 or higher	or	90 or higher
Hypertension Crisis (Consult your doctor immediately)	Higher than 180	and/or	Higher than 120

What is hypertension?

Also known as high blood pressure, this condition occurs when the blood pressure in your arteries rises above what is considered normal.

How common is hypertension?

Among individuals with obesity, nearly half (42%) also have hypertension (Wang and Wang, 2004). Hypertension is quite common; one out of every three American adults carries a diagnosis of hypertension (Merai et al, 2016).

What are the signs and symptoms of hypertension?

Usually hypertension has no symptoms and is detected on a routine blood pressure check. When symptoms are present, they can include headaches, chest pain, vision changes, a general feeling of being unwell, dizziness or lightheadedness, anxiety, or nausea and vomiting. If you are having any serious symptoms, you should call emergency services (9-1-1 in the United States) or proceed to your nearest emergency room.

How is hypertension diagnosed?

Hypertension is diagnosed by elevated blood pressure readings at your doctor's office. You can also check it at your local pharmacy or at home, and you should notify your doctor if you find that you have high blood pressure readings (over 130/80 mm Hg). Doctors use published guidelines to determine whether you have hypertension and how it should be treated. For those aged 60 years or less with no diabetes or chronic kidney disease, the blood pressure should be less than 130/80 mm Hg. For those older than 60 years without diabetes or chronic kidney disease, the goal is less than 130/80 mm Hg. For anyone with diabetes or chronic kidney disease, regardless of age, the blood pressure should be less than 130/80 mm Hg. If your blood pressure readings are higher than these numbers, you will be diagnosed with hypertension.

How is hypertension treated?

Treating hypertension will consist of you making changes at home and taking the medications that your doctor feels are necessary for you to achieve the goals for your blood pressure. Treatment also consists of scheduled visits to have your blood pressure checked. Some medications will require routine bloodwork to monitor your *electrolytes* and kidney function. The changes you can make at home include eating a low-salt diet, along with a diet that is heart- and weight-healthy. Regular exercise, at least 30 minutes per day for 5 days per week, will also help to lower your blood pressure.

Should I learn anything else about hypertension?

It is important to know that hypertension is a risk factor for two other important diseases that we discuss later in this chapter, which are *coronary artery disease* and *cerebrovascular disease*. These terms include what is commonly referred to as *heart attacks (myocardial infarction)* and *strokes*. Preventing hypertension or keeping it well managed will reduce your risk of these complications.

Coronary Artery Disease

What is coronary artery disease (CAD)?

This is when there is a buildup of *plaque*, which contains cholesterol, in the arteries that supply blood to the heart (*coronary arteries*). When the buildup causes severe narrowing (*stenosis*) of an artery, a heart attack can occur due to decreased blood flow to the heart. When blood flow to the arteries that supply the heart becomes inadequate, it can cause a heart attack (myocardial infarction). During a heart attack, the heart muscle does not receive enough oxygen due to a lack of blood flow, and it can be damaged or stop functioning altogether. This damage to the heart can lead to *heart failure*, or possibly death if it is severe.

How common is CAD?

Heart disease is the leading cause of death among American men and women. CAD is the most common type of heart disease, and every year more than 735,000 Americans suffer a heart attack as a result. Roughly 370,000 people die each year due to CAD (CDC Heart Disease Facts, 2017). The importance of these numbers lies in the fact that most of these deaths are preventable. CAD develops over many years due to risk factors as well as genetics. We can prevent or control the risk factors for CAD, which include obesity, high blood pressure, diabetes, and high cholesterol.

What are the symptoms and signs of CAD?

Chest pain is an important symptom. The pain is usually on the left side or the center of the chest. It can be intermittent and mild to moderate, or sudden and severe. Sensations of *heartburn*, left-sided jaw pain, left-arm pain, and upper-abdominal pain are also possible. You might also notice shortness of breath, sweating, dizziness, or lightheadedness. Not everyone with CAD has chest pain; those with diabetes and women tend to present atypically. If you believe that you might have CAD, you should inform your primary-care physician immediately. If you experience symptoms concerning for a heart attack, call emergency services (9-1-1) right away.

How is CAD diagnosed?

Your doctor might order tests (such as an *electrocardiogram* [EKG or ECG], an *echocardiogram* [an ultrasound of your heart], a *stress test*, and/or a *cardiac catheterization* [a procedure in which dye is injected into your heart to see whether the arteries supplying your heart are clogged]) for diagnosis.

How is CAD treated?

What you can do at home to prevent CAD is to eat a heart-healthy diet, keep your weight within the recommended limits, and exercise regularly, as recommended. If you have already been diagnosed with CAD or any of the diseases that are risk factors for CAD, it is still important to focus on what you eat and on your exercise levels as well as on taking all of your medications as prescribed and following-up with you doctors as scheduled. You might be placed on medications such as aspirin, blood-thinners, cholesterol-lowering medications, and other heart medications.

Is there anything else I should know about CAD?

CAD can lead to *congestive heart failure* (CHF), a condition that follows damage to the heart leading to inefficient function. If you or a family member is interested in more information regarding CHF, you can visit https://www.cdc.gov/dhdsp/data_statistics/fact_sheets/fs_heart_failure.htm.

Cerebrovascular Disease

What is cerebrovascular disease?

The most common manifestation of this disorder is a stroke (*cerebrovascular accident* [CVA]). It is like losing blood flow to the heart in a heart attack, but it occurs in the brain, leading to a stroke. Plaques containing cholesterol can build up in the arteries that supply the brain. The plaques can cause severe narrowing of the arteries and a decrease in blood flow to the brain. These plaques can also break off and travel into the smaller arteries and become lodged there, cutting off blood flow to the part of the brain that is supplied by these arteries.

How common is cerebrovascular disease?

Each year, more than 795,000 Americans suffer a stroke, and it is a leading cause of long-term disability in the country (CDC Stroke Facts, 2017).

What are the symptoms and signs of cerebrovascular disease?

The symptoms of a stroke include difficulty speaking or understanding what someone is saying, difficulty moving your arms or legs, facial droop, confusion or decreased alertness, numbness or tingling in your limbs, dizziness, and sudden headache. A *mnemonic* to help remember the main symptoms and what to do when a stroke occurs is F-A-S-T:

F – Face drooping
A – Arm weakness
S – Speech difficulty
T – Time to call 9-1-1

How are strokes diagnosed?

A stroke is diagnosed by assessing symptoms along with the use of *imaging studies* of the brain, which include a *computerized tomography* (CT) *scan*, a *magnetic resonance imaging* (MRI) *scan*, or both.

How are strokes treated?

If you suspect that you or someone you know might be having a stroke, time is of the essence because there is a small window of time in which treatment can be given before permanent damage develops. This treatment consists of medication that can dissolve the clot that is blocking blood flow to the brain. If you are a candidate for it, it can be given only within a few hours of the start of the symptoms. Therefore, as soon as a stroke is suspected, you should call emergency services (9-1-1) immediately to be taken by ambulance to the nearest emergency room.

Is there anything else I should know about strokes?

Following are some additional on-line resources:

National Stroke Association: http://www.stroke.org/

American Stroke Association: http://www.strokeassociation.org/STROKEORG/

Thromboembolic Disease

Given its high mortality rate, *thromboembolic disease* (blood clots in major blood vessels), or *thromboembolism*, is the third most common vascular disease in the United States. *Thromboemboli* can arise from the formation of blood clots in either arteries or veins. In response to blood vessel injuries, blood clots form as clusters of *aggregated platelets* and red blood cells that accumulate at the site of injury; they act as plugs to prevent leakage of the vessels. However, blood clots can negatively affect blood flow by disrupting the directional flow during circulation. These clusters of platelets and red blood cells can leave the injury site and enter a different part of the *circulatory system*; hence, a thromboembolism (What is Deep Vein Thrombosis? 2011). Thromboembolic disease can present in arteries as *arterial thromboembolism*, and in veins as *venous thromboembolism*.

This section focuses on venous thromboembolism (VTE) and its status as a medical complication of obesity. VTE is a chronic vascular disease that involves two clinical conditions: *deep-vein thrombosis* (DVT) and *pulmonary embolism* (PE). DVT is caused by the formation of a blood clot in the veins of the legs or the pelvis. Pulmonary emboli occurs when the blood clot leaves, travels to, and blocks the pulmonary arteries, which aid in the oxygenation of blood in the lungs (Yang, De Staercke, & Hooper, 2012; Stein, Beemath, & Olson, 2005). Symptoms of VTE can range from swelling and pain to cardiac and respiratory failure and death, especially if untreated. Although VTE is considered a dangerous yet preventable disease, recent findings from a 2015 survey highlighted a relative lack of global public awareness of VTE and its associations with stroke and heart disease (Wendelboe et al, 2015). With the rising rates of obesity, it is important to improve our understanding of VTE and its link to obesity as a moderate risk factor. Studies have shown that a high BMI correlates with an increased risk of VTE (Yang et al, 2012). Additionally, obesity interacts with risk factors associated with VTE. For example, excess fat tissue in those with obesity can cause *hypoxia* (a decrease in oxygenation) and indirectly increases the synthesis of *coagulation factors* (factors that cause the blood to clot) in the circulatory system (Yang et al, 2012). An increase in coagulation can lead to more blood clots in the system. These indirect interactions between obesity (high amounts of fat tissue) and VTE can lead to PE, which are primary contributors to higher mortality rates of VTE.

Heart Disease

As the leading cause of death in the United States, heart disease is common in many Americans. According to the CDC, 610,000 people die from heart disease each year, which is a fatality rate of 1 in 4 Americans (Heart Disease Facts, 2017). As shown in Table 6-2, heart disease is also the leading cause of death for Americans of most race/ethnic groups.

Table 6-2: Percentage of Deaths Caused by Heart Disease in 2008 for Different Races (Source: Heart Disease Facts, 2017)

Race of Ethnic Group	% of Deaths
American Indians or Alaska Natives	18.4
Asians or Pacific Islanders	22.2
Non-Hispanic Blacks	23.8
Non-Hispanic Whites	23.8
All	23.5

This section focuses on the various heart conditions that fall under the umbrella of heart disease that can complicate overweight or obesity. These conditions involve a narrowing or blocking of the blood vessels that surround the heart (Figure 6-1), in addition to defects in the muscle, valves, or rhythm of the heart. Although some forms of heart disease can be caused by family genetics, other forms, such as CAD, can be caused by a poor diet and by a lack of physical activity, both being risk factors for obesity. CAD is the most common form of heart disease; 16.5 million Americans aged 20 years or older have the disease, and more than 370,000 people die from CAD each year (Heart Disease Facts, 2017; Wilson & Douglas, 2016). It is described as having blockages in the coronary arteries. Blocking blood flow in coronary arteries affects the level of oxygen that the heart muscle receive. When not enough oxygenated blood is pumped throughout the heart muscle, a fatal heart attack can occur.

Because we now know that heart disease is caused by the narrowing or blockage of a coronary artery, let's dive deeper in understanding how these blockages occur. According to the National Health and Nutrition Examination Survey (NHANES) and the CDC, approximately half of American adults have at least one of three major risk factors for CAD, including hypertension (high blood pressure), high cholesterol, or cigarette smoking (Heart Disease Facts, 2017; Fryar et al, 2012). As stated in the section "Hypertension" earlier in the chapter, diets high in salt and cholesterol can contribute to high blood pressure, which can lead to further blockages of blood vessels. In tandem with the plaque buildup from cigarette smoking, these three factors can lead to untoward physical changes in a person's body weight. Other risk factors for heart disease include diabetes mellitus, alcoholism, a poor diet, and a sedentary lifestyle (Heart Disease Facts, 2017). Because having these conditions intensifies their association with overweight or obesity, they simultaneously increase the risk of CAD or other forms of heart disease (narrowing arteries) as potential complications (Heart Disease Facts, 2017; Wilson & Douglas, 2016; Fryar et al, 2012).

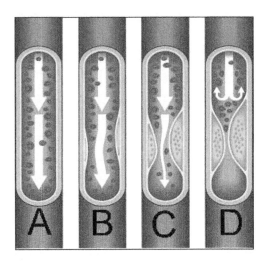

Figure 6-1: A) An artery with normal blood flow. D) An artery with a buildup of plaque, causing blockage of blood flow, which can lead to CAD. (Source: Heart Disease Facts, 2017)

The influence of overweight and obesity on heart disease has been further examined in studies that have verified the link between the BMI of people with overweight and obesity and the risk factors for heart failure and disease. Results from these studies have confirmed correlations between a higher BMI and an increase in the likelihood that one will develop heart failure. Specifically, obesity was linked to defects in the heart muscle, as the muscle tissue increased in size due to higher blood pressures needed by the heart to pump blood (Kenchaiah et al, 2002). As the BMI of people enters into classes of overweight and obesity (BMI: 25–29.9 [overweight]; 30–34.9 [Class I obesity: mild]; 35–39.9 [Class II obesity: moderate]; ≥40 [Class III obesity: severe]), their risk of heart disease dramatically increases. Unfortunately, the risk of heart disease is associated with many conditions (e.g., hypertension, sleep apnea, type 2 diabetes mellitus), which we cover next.

Which Pulmonary Conditions Are Worsened by Obesity?

Sleep Apnea

Sleep apnea is a chronic sleep disorder marked by repeated awakenings during a person's sleep. There are three types of sleep apnea: obstructive, central, and complex (Sleep Apnea, 2015). *Obstructive sleep apnea* (OSA) is caused by the relaxation of throat muscles, which obstruct the breathing pathway during sleep. *Central sleep apnea* is caused by the brain's inability to send signals to the muscles that control breathing. *Complex (or mixed) sleep apnea* is a combination of obstructive and central sleep apnea (Sleep Apnea, 2015; Strohl, 2016). OSA is the most common type of sleep-related breathing disorder. It is considered a serious condition due to its complications, which include an increased risk of heart disease and hypertension. OSA can range from mild, moderate, to severe, based on the number of loss-of-breathing (*apneic*) episodes that a person experiences. Currently, nearly half (45%) of adults and children (46%) with obesity suffer from OSA (Romero-Corral et al, 2010). Like hypertension, obesity is a *risk factor* for OSA given that the *prevalence* of OSA increases with higher BMI values of obesity (Strohl, 2016; Romero-Corral et al, 2010).

The relationship between OSA and obesity is complex. The increased fat tissue that is present in those with obesity can surround and disrupt the breathing pathways, leading to OSA. However, complications of OSA, such as increased appetite and decreased energy levels, can be driving factors for developing obesity (Romero-Corral et al, 2010). *Genetic factors* are suggested to influence the interaction between both conditions. Further studies can provide more conclusive evidence on the cause-and-effect relationship between OSA and obesity. In terms of treating OSA, *continuous positive airway pressure* (CPAP) therapy is the most common treatment. CPAP therapy requires that those with OSA be attached to a *ventilator* (breathing machine) while they are asleep; this device applies air under pressure and keeps the breathing pathways open while the person is sleeping. Weight loss and *bariatric surgery* in those with obesity and OSA has also been effective in reducing the severity of OSA; this often leads to the reduction of other risk factors (Strohl, 2016; Romero-Corral et al, 2010).

OSA

What is OSA?

OSA is a breathing disorder that occurs during sleep, and it can cause you to stop breathing (apnea) episodically while you sleep. Obstruction in the back of your throat is the underlying cause, and this occurs more in people with obesity because they tend to have more tissue in the back of their throats. When the tissues in the throat relax during sleep, the airway becomes blocked. There can be other reasons for obstructions in the throat (such as enlarged tonsils and adenoids); however, obesity is the most common cause of sleep apnea in adults.

How common is OSA?

OSA is estimated to affect 3% to 7% of adults in the United States (Punjabi, 2008) and approximately 1% to 4% of children (Lumeng and Chervin, 2008).

What are the symptoms and signs of OSA?

OSA is suspected when you have a combination of the following symptoms or signs: snoring, insomnia, fatigue or daytime napping, high blood pressure or high blood counts (*hemoglobin* and *hematocrit*), a large neck size (shirt collar greater than 16 inches), a large tongue, or apnea (if someone has noticed that you stop breathing intermittently while sleeping). You might also experience waking up and choking, snorting, coughing, or gasping for air. When there is decreased oxygen to the lungs, the heart compensates by working harder to deliver more blood to the body. This in turn can lead to high blood pressure.

How is OSA diagnosed?

The diagnosis is made with a sleep study, called a *polysomnogram*, that can be ordered by your primary-care physician. During this test, you are monitored overnight for signs of OSA.

How is OSA treated?

If obesity is a cause of your OSA, weight loss will be part of your treatment plan, and it might be a solution, because OSA can be reversed. As long as you have OSA, you might need to use a sleep machine such as the aforementioned CPAP or a *Bilevel Positive Airway Pressure* (BiPAP) machine during sleep. This machine pushes air into and/or out of your lungs to help them expand fully. It is important to supply oxygen to, and remove carbon dioxide from, the blood. Addressing your weight as an underlying factor for OSA is key because this can reverse OSA.

Is there anything else I should know about OSA?

If OSA is left untreated, it can lead to high blood pressure and an elevated heart rate, which can place excess strain on the heart. Over time, the increased work load on the heart can lead to heart failure. OSA can also lead to a higher risk of CAD, stroke, diabetes, and premature death. The lungs can also be strained, leading to a condition called *pulmonary hypertension* (increased pressure in the *pulmonary arteries*), which can also lead to heart failure.

Obesity Hypoventilation Syndrome

What is obesity hypoventilation syndrome (OHS)?

Also known as *Pickwickian syndrome*, this is a disease in which the excess weight on the outside of the body restricts the lungs from expanding completely. When the lungs cannot expand completely, they cannot perform the function of exchanging oxygen and carbon dioxide effectively. This leads to an accumulation of carbon dioxide and a decrease in oxygen supply to the blood.

What are the symptoms and signs of OHS?

Fatigue, loss of energy, shortness of breath, daytime sleepiness, snoring while sleeping, or pauses in breathing can be present.

How is OHS diagnosed?

If you feel that you might have OHS, you should be evaluated by your doctor. Your doctor will likely want to know about your sleeping habits as well as the levels of oxygen and carbon dioxide in your blood. A polysomnogram might also be ordered.

How is OHS treated?

As is the case with OSA, weight loss is key. CPAP or BiPAP machines might also be used to ensure an adequate oxygen supply and carbon dioxide removal.

Is there anything else I should know about OHS?

Is it important to know if you have OSA or OHS because they can be risk factors for complications during procedures or surgeries that require anesthesia. You might need more assistance with breathing during or after surgical procedures.

Which Endocrine/Metabolic Conditions Are Worsened by Obesity?

Type 2 Diabetes Mellitus

What is type 2 diabetes mellitus? Type 2 diabetes mellitus occurs when the body becomes resistant to the effects of *insulin*. Insulin is the *hormone* that our body produces to reduce levels of *glucose* (sugar) in our blood. It usually works on the muscles and other tissues in the body to help them utilize the sugar circulating in the blood. Fat buildup in the blood causes resistance to the effects of insulin, and then the tissues cannot take sugar out of the blood like they are supposed to, which leads to high sugar levels in the blood. Over time, uncontrolled high sugar levels in the blood can damage the circulatory system, which can contribute to vision loss, heart attacks, strokes, limb loss, and damage to the kidneys and nerves. It also affects the immune system, leading to more frequent infections and impairments in healing after injuries.

How common is type 2 diabetes?

Type 2 diabetes is a disease of obesity, and as such, rates have increased along with obesity rates in the United States. Type 2 diabetes is very common, effecting more than 29 million people in the United States, and an estimated 422 million people globally! (National Center for Chronic Diseases, 2017; WHO, 2017).

What are the symptoms and signs of type 2 diabetes?

Symptoms of diabetes include increased thirst, increased urinary frequency, and increased amount of urine production.

How is type 2 diabetes diagnosed?

In your blood work, an *HbA1C* level greater than 6.5% or a fasting blood sugar level greater than 126 on two separate occasions is used to diagnose diabetes.

How is type 2 diabetes treated?

Depending on your blood sugar levels, your doctor might treat you with diet and exercise, or this combination along with (oral or injectable) medications and/or insulin. You will also be placed on a baby aspirin each day, as a preventive measure against cardiovascular disease. Your doctor will likely add an *angiotensin-converting enzyme* (ACE) *inhibitor* or *angiotensin II receptor blocker* (ARB) medication to your regimen. These are blood pressure medications, but they are also given to people with diabetes to help protect their kidneys. If your cholesterol is high, your doctor will start you on a medicine to help lower your cholesterol (generally a medication known as a *statin*). You might not receive some of these medications if you are not able to take them for specific reasons.

Is there anything else I should know about type 2 diabetes?

Keep in mind that it is the high blood sugar levels in diabetes that cause the damage. If you are already a diabetic, don't worry! The key is to prevent the complications of diabetes. You can do this by keeping your blood sugar levels within the recommended levels. And, you can achieve this by taking your medicines as prescribed, following a diabetic diet, exercising regularly, and following up with your doctor to ensure that you are being monitored for any of the aforementioned complications.

Diabetes doesn't develop overnight, Rather, it usually takes many years to develop. The good thing about this is that you can prevent it by tackling the issues that lead to obesity. If you already have diabetes, there are measures that you can take to improve or reverse it if you are in the early stages. If you think that you might have diabetes, make an appointment with your doctor and be sure to express your concerns.

Hyperlipidemia

What is hyperlipidemia?

This is when there is elevated cholesterol or *triglycerides* in the blood.

How common is hyperlipidemia?

It is very common; more than 73.5 million American adults have *elevated low-density lipoprotein* (LDL, the "bad cholesterol") levels.

What are the symptoms and signs of hyperlipidemia?

Usually there are none. High cholesterol is usually found on routine blood work; however, if cholesterol levels are severely elevated, there can be physical manifestations due to fatty deposits in the body, especially when the cholesterol level is greatly elevated. These deposits or physical manifestations include *xanthomas* or *xanthelasmas*.

How is hyperlipidemia diagnosed?

It is diagnosed with blood work, specifically a *lipid panel* that is ordered by your doctor. The lipid panel will show the levels of different fats in your blood, including total cholesterol, *high-density lipoprotein* (HDL, or "good cholesterol"), LDL, and triglycerides. Adults who have not been diagnosed with hyperlipidemia should still have their levels checked at least once every 5 years.

How is hyperlipidemia treated?

Your doctor will determine the right treatment for you based on your risk factors. If you don't have many risk factors, your doctor might try a trial of diet and exercise to bring your cholesterol levels down. If your doctor recommends a prescription medication, you should still continue a good diet and exercise regimen. The first-line medication for high cholesterol and triglycerides is a statin medication. If you are already on a statin medication, your doctor might be following your cholesterol closely to see whether you need adjustments in your dose. If you cannot tolerate a statin for any reason, there are alternative medications that your doctor can prescribe. If you have high triglycerides only, your doctor might also recommend fish-oil supplements. You should check with your doctor before starting any over-the-counter medications because they could interfere with your prescription medications.

Is there anything else I should know about hyperlipidemia?

The most important thing to know about hyperlipidemia is that it is a risk factor and contributor to several other conditions such as heart attacks and strokes. If you have a strong family history of hyperlipidemia, you should inform your doctor so that he or she can check your lipids and monitor you more closely.

Metabolic Syndrome

Metabolic syndrome is not an individual disease. Rather, it is a collection of the following diseases: hypertension, high blood glucose levels, elevated cholesterol levels, and obesity (specifically excess weight around the waist). This syndrome is important because having this collection of diseases significantly increases your risk of heart attacks and strokes.

Type 2 Diabetes Mellitus

Like heart disease, diabetes mellitus (usually shortened to diabetes) is a common and chronic condition that affects many Americans; it is often considered one of the most challenging complications of obesity. When the term "diabetes mellitus" is broken down, "diabetes" in Greek means "to pass through," and "mellitus" in Latin means "sweet," which accurately describes the "high sugar" levels in the blood associated with diabetes. Diabetes mellitus involves the dysfunctional interaction between our bodies and the insulin hormone during digestion. When we ingest and process food, our bodies break down the food into glucose (sugar) molecules, which are vital energy sources for our organs, tissues, and cells. An organ called the *pancreas*, which lies adjacent to the stomach, produces and releases insulin into the bloodstream in the presence of glucose. Insulin signals cells in the body to absorb the glucose molecules produced by food breakdown, which is used for energy (Diabetes, 2017). People with diabetes have difficulty producing or releasing insulin, causing glucose to stay in the bloodstream, yielding high blood glucose (sugar) levels. The two most common types of diabetes are type 1 and type 2 diabetes mellitus. *Type 1 diabetes* involves the body's *immune system*, which is responsible for protecting the body from foreign pathogens; in this condition, the body attacks its own pancreas cells that produce insulin. This results in the body's inability to make insulin, leading to high blood sugar levels. Type 1 diabetes is usually diagnosed early in life, in children and adolescents, and requires insulin injections to maintain proper glucose levels (What is Diabetes? 2016).

Type 2 diabetes, the obesity complication we are focusing on here, accounts for most of the diagnosed diabetes cases in the United States. It can be acquired during childhood or adulthood. The cells in the person with type 2 diabetes resist the effects of insulin, leading to a failure to absorb or store glucose. This inability can cause increased glucose levels in the bloodstream, which increases the demand for more insulin to be produced by the pancreas. Eventually, insulin-producing cells become exhausted, leading to an overall decreased amount of insulin released (Diabetes, 2017; What is Diabetes? 2016). Figure 6-2 further depicts this interaction. Diagnoses for type 2 diabetes and *pre-diabetes* (the precursor stage of type 2 diabetes) are made through either a *fasting* or *random blood glucose* (sugar) test, which measures the glucose concentration from a drawn blood sample. A fasting glucose test is typically done in the morning on an empty stomach (that is, without having eaten), whereas a random glucose test can be done at any time during the day (Diabetes, 2017). Blood glucose (sugar) level readings are read in milligrams per deciliter (*mg/dL*) and can indicate type 2 diabetes (≥126 mg/dL in a fasting sample, or 200 mg/dL in a random sample), pre-diabetes (100–125 mg/dL on a fasting test or 140–200 mg/dL on a random test), or normal levels (<100 mg/dL on a fasting test or <140 mg/dL on a random test) (Managing Diabetes, 2017). Additionally, a *hemoglobin A1C* lab test is given to those with diabetes two to four times each year to determine how effectively people are managing their condition. The A1C test can measure your average blood glucose (sugar) levels for the past 2 to 3 months. Specifically, this test measures the amount of glucose that attaches to the hemoglobin molecules of red blood cells. The A1C levels can be associated with a diagnosis of type 2 diabetes (6.5% or higher) or pre-diabetes (5.7%–6.4%). Therefore, the higher the A1C levels, the higher the glucose levels are in both the bloodstream and in the hemoglobin (Managing Diabetes, 2017).

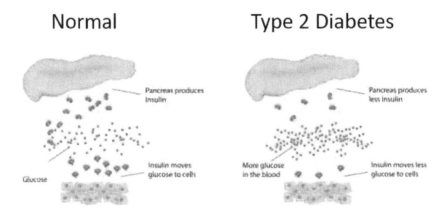

Figure 6-2: Comparison of the pancreas as normal versus with type 2 diabetes. The loss of function in producing adequate levels of insulin by the pancreas (type 2 diabetes) causes more glucose in the bloodstream (Type 2 diabetes, 2017).

Pre-diabetes and type 2 diabetes are chronic conditions that affect more than 11% of Americans aged 20 years or older (Eckel et al, 2011). Non-variable factors (e.g., race, age, genetics) can affect the likelihood that a person will develop type 2 diabetes, but poor habits (e.g., an unhealthy diet, inadequate physical exercise) are major contributors, as well. Excess weight (with a high BMI) is an established risk factor for type 2 diabetes, given that an increase in fat tissue can result in the insulin resistance that is common in those with diabetes. Although there is currently no cure for this condition, researchers have been able to understand more fully the exact mechanisms involved in both type 2 diabetes and obesity. The excess *adipose* (fat) tissues in patients with overweight or obesity release certain hormones and proteins that directly induce their bodies' cells to be resistant to insulin. This resistance can then contribute to the decreased uptake of glucose by those cells (Eckel et al, 2011; Kahn et al, 2006). Common symptoms associated with type 2 diabetes include frequent thirst and urination, fatigue, numbness in the hands and feet, blurry vision, and an inability to heal wounds properly (Managing Diabetes, 2017). These symptoms negatively affect a person's quality of life.

Fortunately, lifestyle changes (e.g., healthy diet, increased exercise), insulin therapy, taking prescribed medications, and weight-loss surgery are proven to be effective in preventing, managing, and even reversing the insulin resistance/type 2 diabetes associated with obesity. Early detection and immediate management can greatly reduce the negative impact of these chronic conditions, in addition to preventing further development of health issues associated with obesity and type 2 diabetes (such as heart disease and strokes). For patients with *refractory*, or unmanageable, type 2 diabetes, weight-loss surgery is the best tactic for improved glucose control or for complete remission of the disease (Surgery for Diabetes, 2017).

Which Musculoskeletal Conditions Are Worsened by Obesity?

Arthritis

The progression of arthritis in patients with overweight and obesity is common. Although this major obesity comorbidity is prevalent, *arthritis* is not well understood by the public. There are multiple types of arthritic conditions, but arthritis is generally defined as *inflammation* (swelling) and pain in the joints (i.e., the spaces between bones). In this section, we focus on *osteoarthritis*. Osteoarthritis is the most common type of arthritis, affecting more than 30 million adults in the United States (Zhang and Jordan, 2010). The prevalence of symptomatic osteoarthritis can vary based on the specific joint (e.g., the knee, hand, hip) studied, but prevalence rates will likely increase due to the obesity epidemic. Globally, 10% of men and 18% of women older than age 60 suffer from osteoarthritis (Zhang and Jordan, 2010).

Osteoarthritis is characterized by the degradation of cartilage, the layer of tissue that lines the joints of our bones. As the cartilage within joints break down, the bones between the joints rub against each other; this can lead to pain and inflammation (Kane, 2017). Osteoarthritis can be caused by increased stress placed on the joints, creating consistent wear-and-tear damage in the cartilage. Excess weight associated with obesity might play a role in the increased stress within joints that leads to osteoarthritis. In American adults with arthritis, obesity is 54% more prevalent compared to adults without arthritis, resulting in a positive association between a high BMI and arthritis (Kane, 2017; Hottman et al, 2011). Each pound obtained from excess weight can provide an extra four pounds of pressure in major joints, like the hips and the knees (Kane, 2017). The pressure and arthritic pain placed in knees and hips of patients with overweight or obesity can lead to a need for surgical replacement of these joints (to improve function and alleviate pain). Due to the increased sensitivity in arthritic-induced strained joints, health-care providers typically advise strength-building physical therapy for patients with both conditions, to properly promote joint health and weight loss. Arthritis can be a difficult barrier to overcome for those with obesity. An individualized and properly managed weight-loss approach allows you to take significant steps to overcome both chronic conditions.

Osteoarthritis

What is osteoarthritis?

This is a type or chronic arthritis that develops after long periods of wear and tear or trauma to the cartilage (a type of tissue) in the joints. Commonly involved areas are the back and knees. Excess body weight will place an excess load on many joints of the body. If your joints are holding more weight than they were designed to, this will lead to eventual wear and tear in the long run.

How common is osteoarthritis?

Osteoarthritis is the most common joint disorder in the United States. It affects 10% of men and 13% of women ages 60 and older.

What are the symptoms or signs of osteoarthritis?

You might have chronic pain in the affected joint, that can be worse when you use that joint more. Sometimes, there is swelling of the joint and difficulty moving it due to pain or stiffness.

How is osteoarthritis diagnosed?

It is usually diagnosed by symptoms along with X-rays.

How is osteoarthritis treated?

Osteoarthritis is not reversible, so controlling pain from the disease and preventing further damage are the main focus of treatment. Pain control is a step-up therapy and is individualized to each person. Pain control usually involves several different therapies including rest, heat or ice, physical therapy, topical agents, over-the-counter analgesics or anti-inflammatory medications, or prescription pain medications. When osteoarthritis is severe and debilitating, your doctor might refer you to an orthopedist for *steroids* or *hyaluronic acid injections* into the joint, or for joint replacement surgery. Preventing further injury is the goal of the exercise that you will do to lose weight; this will also help your joints strengthen and improve your mobility, so it's more reason to put on your exercise gear and get going!

Gout

As you just read in the previous section, osteoarthritis is described as a condition characterized by the degradation of cartilage that lines one's joints. Another type of arthritis is *inflammatory arthritis*, which is marked by inflammation of the joints, which leads to pain, swelling, and stiffness. *Gout* is one type of inflammatory arthritis, and it is the most common form of inflammatory arthritis in adult men in the United States (Cho et al, 2005). According to a 2007–2008 NHANES report, approximately 4% of American adults have gout, with a significantly higher incidence and prevalence found in men as compared to women (Kuo et al, 2015). Gout is caused by elevated levels of *uric acid* in the bloodstream, which can lead to the formation and accumulation of uric acid crystals in the joint spaces. The presence of uric acid crystals in joints can trigger painful inflammatory attacks, which can be worse for people with overweight or obesity.

To understand how gout attacks occur, we must understand the disease and its association with obesity. Uric acid is a byproduct of the breakdown of purine compounds in the liver (Choi et al, 2005). Purine compounds are either synthesized naturally in the body or ingested in our food. They are found in high concentrations in specific meats and seafood. Thus, diets high in meat and seafood are often associated with high uric acid concentrations in the bloodstream. Normally, uric acid is filtered by the kidneys and excreted through the urine. However, excess adipose (fat) tissue can slow down the filtration of uric acid by the kidneys, elevating uric acid levels in the bloodstream and potentially causing gout attacks (Kane, 2017; Choi et al, 2005).

Excess weight can also cause kidney dysfunction due to its role in insulin production. As mentioned in the section "Type 2 Diabetes Mellitus" earlier in the chapter, excess weight can induce insulin resistance in the body's cells, which leads to elevated levels of both blood glucose and insulin levels (Kahn et al, 2006). The high levels of insulin in the circulation inhibit the proper filtration and excretion of uric acid by the kidneys (Becker, 2016). In summary, excess adipose (fat) tissue in the body due to overweight or obesity plays an important role in insulin resistance, which indirectly leads to high uric acid levels and to the presentation of gout. Thus, it is important to identify and treat any of the underlying conditions (obesity or type 2 diabetes) that might contribute to the gout attacks (Becker, 2016).

What is gout?

Gout is also a type of arthritis, but it is different from osteoarthritis in many ways. The mechanism behind gout involves formation and deposit of uric acid crystals into the joints. Uric acid is the product of the breakdown of purines in the body. Purines are found in high amounts in organ meats, red meats, and seafood, which are consumed in higher amounts in Western diets. Alcohol, especially beer, also raises uric acid levels in the blood, and this also tends to be consumed in higher amounts in the Western diet. Therefore, obese patients have a higher incidence of gout. The first joint often affected is the big toe, a condition called *podagra*. Other commonly affected joints include the elbows and knees.

What are the symptoms and signs of gout?

Gout usually presents as acute episodes called gout flares or "attacks" in which there is redness, increased warmth, swelling, and significant pain in one or more joints. The most commonly affected joints are in the toes, other joints in the foot, ankles, knees, and elbows. The pain can cause inability to use the joint.

How is gout treated?

You should avoid foods that can lead to gout (organ meats, red meats, and seafood), and alcohol as much as possible. Changing your diet can prevent gout attacks, and this should be something you do along with taking medications that your doctor recommends. Your doctor will prescribe certain *anti-inflammatory medications* or a steroid injection into the affected joint during a flare. If you have more than a few attacks a year, your doctor will put you on a daily maintenance medication to prevent future gout flares. This is important because recurrent gout flares can damage the joints and lead to chronic arthritis and pain. If you experience what you believe is a gout flare, you should see a doctor immediately to first make sure it is gout and to get treatment quickly. Another condition, called *septic arthritis* (infection of a joint), can look like gout, but have serious consequences if it is not recognized promptly.

Which Gastrointestinal Conditions Are Worsened by Obesity?

Cholelithiasis

What is cholelithiasis?

This is when *gallstones* form in the biliary system (organs and ducts that make, store, and secrete bile). The part of the biliary system they most commonly form in is the gallbladder, which is an organ located just under the liver. Obesity significantly increases the risk of developing cholelithiasis. Gallstones are partially made of cholesterol, and obesity increases the formation of them.

How common are gallstones?

It is estimated that about 20 million adults (Everhart & Ruhl, 2009) and about 2% of children (Wesdorp et al, 2000) in the United States have cholelithiasis.

What are the symptoms and signs of gallbladder disease?

Gallstones often sit undetected. When a gallstone causes inflammation of the gallbladder or blocks the duct that leads out of the gallbladder, it can lead to symptoms, such as upper-right or middle abdominal pain, nausea, and/or vomiting. This pain can be noticeably worse after eating. If you notice symptoms like these, make an appointment with your doctor immediately. If your symptoms are severe, or you cannot keep food or water down, go to the emergency room immediately.

How are gallstones diagnosed?

Gallstones can be diagnosed with an ultrasound of your gallbladder. If gallstones are not clearly seen on the ultrasound, further testing, such as with a *hepatobiliary iminodiacetic acid* (HIDA) *scan*, might be needed.

How are gallstones treated?

Treatment will depend on the level of disease you have as well as whether the gallstones are causing symptoms. If the gallstones are not causing symptoms, your doctor will likely opt for routine follow-up and monitoring of symptoms. If the gallstones are causing symptoms, you will likely need your gallbladder removed by a surgical procedure, called a *cholecystectomy.*

Is there anything else I should know about gallbladder disease?

When cholelithiasis leads to inflammation of the gallbladder, it is called *cholecystitis.* Cholecystitis is a condition that requires urgent evaluation and treatment, which can include medications and/or surgery. Cholelithiasis is also a risk for *pancreatitis*, which is an acute inflammation of the pancreas.

Non-Alcoholic Fatty Liver Disease

The *liver*, one of the largest organs in the body, is responsible for the metabolic break-down of nutrients such as fat (fatty acids), carbohydrates, and proteins. The liver also receives toxic substances from the blood and detoxifies them into harmless substances that can properly be excreted from the body. Abnormalities in the liver's metabolic functions can lead to a variety of conditions, including *non-alcoholic fatty liver disease* (NAFLD). NAFLD is characterized by a buildup of extra fat in liver cells due to the liver's difficulty in breaking down those fats. A diagnosis of NAFLD is made when up to 10% of the liver's weight is composed of fat. When the rate of fat uptake is greater than the rate of fat breakdown and release by liver cells, fats accumulate and cause abnormalities in the metabolic functions of the liver (Fabbrini et al, 2010).

NAFLD is the most common chronic liver condition in the United States, and it is highly influenced by excess weight and by a high BMI (Fabbrini et al, 2010). Recent studies reveal that NAFLD affects nearly one-third (30%) of the general population of Western nations. NAFLD occurs in every age and race group, but it is more commonly found in middle-aged men (40–50 years old) with overweight/obesity. Rates of NAFLD are also higher in African-Americans (48.3%) compared to rates in Caucasians (32.1%) and Hispanics (17.5%) (Le et al, 2017; Lopez-Velazquez et al, 2014). Although persons with NAFLD often lack prominent symptoms, the chronic condition is associated with a high mortality rate due to its associated risk factors, such as *cirrhosis* of the liver (permanent damage to liver cells), coronary artery disease (CAD), and type 2 diabetes (*insulin resistance*).

NAFLD is exacerbated in those with overweight or obesity. We know that obesity is notable for excess adipose tissue throughout the body. This excess fat tissue releases extra fatty acid molecules that trigger an increased uptake of fat into the liver (Fabbrini et al, 2010). An increase in liver fat contributes to defects in fat metabolism, which leads to fat accumulation (NAFLD) and other adverse medical consequences. Like many of the complications previously discussed, NAFLD is treated by targeting the underlying disease, which is obesity, through therapies (e.g., eating a healthy diet, exercising regularly, taking prescribed weight-loss medications, undergoing weight-loss surgery [the most effective for the treatment of severe obesity]) that lead to weight loss (Sasaki et al, 2014).

What is NAFLD?

NAFLD is what develops when fat builds up in the liver without any relationship to alcohol.

How common is NAFLD?

It is very common, estimated to affect nearly 30% of adults in the United States and nearly 80% to 90% of adults with obesity. NAFLD is reported to be as high as 70% in children with obesity (Bellentani et al, 2010).

What are the symptoms and signs of NAFLD?

There might be none early in the disease. Sometimes, people feel pain in the upper-right side of their abdomen, and your doctor might feel that your liver is large. In advanced stages, you can have yellowing of the skin or eyes (known as *jaundice*), swelling in your abdomen or legs, fatigue, and breast enlargement (in men).

How is NAFLD diagnosed?

Because there are usually no symptoms, the condition might first be suspected through abnormalities of liver tests on routine blood work. These abnormalities will prompt your doctor to order further tests, which will include an ultrasound of your liver. Other tests might follow, including more blood work, or further imaging with a CT scan, MRI scan, or more advanced testing. If these tests do not help to make the diagnosis, a *liver biopsy* might be needed.

How is NAFLD treated?

Treatment will depend on the stage of your disease. Weight loss is recommended if you are overweight or obese. You will also need to protect your liver from harmful substances such as alcohol. Your doctor will recommend medication if you need it for treatment of high cholesterol levels or diabetes, which can contribute to NAFLD. If you are in advanced stages of the disease, you might need a *liver transplant*.

Is there anything else I should know about NAFLD?

NAFLD can lead to non-alcoholic steatohepatitis (*NASH*) (i.e., inflammation of the liver), cirrhosis (permanent damage to the liver leading to dysfunction), or *hepatocellular carcinoma* (liver cancer).

Gastroesophageal Reflux Disease

Gastroesophageal reflux disease (GERD) is a naturally occurring process in which the gastric content from the esophagus is regurgitated back into the esophagus (food pipe), as shown in Figure 6-3 (Marks, 2017). As a brief review, the esophagus and stomach are part of the *digestive system*. Normally, chewed food travels down from the throat to the muscular esophageal tube into the stomach, which releases an acidic solution of gastric juice that aids in food digestion. Although gastroesophageal reflux is a normal process, it becomes a disease (GERD) when the reflux occurs regularly, causing damage to the esophageal lining and producing a painful burning feeling in the chest that is typically called *heartburn* (Definition & Facts for GER and GERD, 2017).

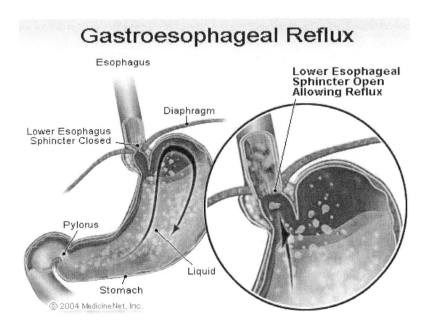

Figure 6-3: Depiction of gastroesophageal reflux; gastric juices from stomach flow back into the esophagus (Marks, 2017).

GERD is a chronic digestive disease that is diagnosed in approximately 20% of the United States population, with a similarly high prevalence in both white and black races (Definition & Facts for GER and GERD, 2017). GERD greatly affects a person's quality of life due to the persistent irritation and reflux that can occur after every meal, with feelings of heartburn lasting from minutes to hours. GERD is also a potential co-morbidity for those with overweight or obesity. Persons with an increased distribution of adipose tissue around their abdomen have an increased likelihood of having GERD because the surrounding body fat can increase the pressure on the stomach, which can lead to movement of the stomach's contents into the esophagus (Kahrilas, 2016). Recent studies have also demonstrated that weight gain, even in normal-weight individuals, increased the likelihood of GERD, regardless of one's BMI (El-Serag, 2008). Continuous heartburn and acid reflux into the esophagus can lead to other conditions, such as the development of ulcers (holes in the digestive lining) and esophageal cancer. Like many of the complications previously discussed, the causal relationship between obesity and GERD suggests that treatments that target both chronic conditions (e.g., behavioral changes, weight-loss surgery) will be effective (Kahrilas, 2016; El-Serag, 2008; El-Hadi, 2014).

What is GERD?

More commonly known as "heartburn," this is when there is reflux of the contents of the stomach, including acid traveling back into the esophagus. Obesity and the so-called "Western diet" are the main causes of this disease.

How common is GERD?

Heartburn is a very common complaint at the doctor's office. GERD is thought to be linked to Western diets, as is obesity, and many obese patients experience GERD. It affects approximately 18% to 28% of the adult population in the United States (El Seraj et al, 2014).

What are the symptoms and signs of GERD?

Symptoms can include a burning sensation in your chest or throat, a sour taste or sensation that there is something in the back of your mouth, coughing (without producing phlegm), hoarse voice, sore throat, feeling acid or food coming up into your mouth, difficulty or discomfort with swallowing.

How is GERD diagnosed?

Your doctor will usually diagnose GERD based on your symptoms. The doctor might do a trial of antacid medications to see whether they improve your symptoms. Occasionally, further testing is needed for a diagnosis, such as a *pH* monitoring test or an *esophagogastroduodenoscopy* (EGD or upper endoscopy).

What is the treatment for GERD?

Because GERD is related to the "Western diet" and lifestyle, changing these are of utmost importance in the treatment and cure of this disease. These changes include avoiding caffeine, alcohol, greasy foods, and any other foods that trigger heartburn for you. Keeping a food diary can help you identify these foods. You should try to lose weight, eat small meals, avoid eating at least a few hours before bedtime, and avoid laying down after meals. Treatment will depend on your symptoms and can consist of a step-up treatment from common fast-acting antacids, to histamine (H_2) blockers, to *proton pump inhibitors.* These are all available over the counter in some form now; however, you might need a prescription-strength medication to control your symptoms. It is important to follow-up with your doctor to make sure your symptoms are controlled and that you do not need further testing.

Is there anything else I should know about GERD?

Smoking also contributes to GERD, so if you're a smoker, this is another reason for you to quit. GERD is important to recognize and treat because untreated, it leads to the esophagus being exposed to the acid from the stomach for long periods of time, which can lead to pre-cancerous changes in the *esophagus*. This is called *Barrett's esophagus*, which requires regular follow-up with EGDs to make sure there isn't progression to cancer.

Which Oncologic (Cancer) Conditions Are Linked with Obesity?

The word cancer can strike us with fear, and most of us probably know someone who has had cancer. It is important to know that although obesity is a risk factor for many cancers there are many other contributors, including tobacco use, alcohol use, genetics, and more. The best thing you can do is cut down on the risk factors that you can control.

To go into the details of each of the cancers that obesity is linked to is beyond the scope of this book. It is, however, important to note the significant link between obesity and cancer and understand that excess fat in the body can influence cancer growth. Table 6-3 presents a chart that lists some of the known cancers linked to obesity.

Table 6-3: Cancerous Conditions Linked to Obesity

Gynecological/ Reproductive	Breast	Endometrial	Ovarian	Cervical	Uterine
Gastrointestinal Tract	Esophageal	Hepatic/Liver	Gallbladder	Pancreatic	Colon
Urinary	Renal				
Other	Prostate				

Endometrial Cancer

In the female human body, the *uterus* (womb) is the reproductive organ located in the pelvic cavity. The uterus receives a fertilized egg that later develops into a fetus, which exits the womb through the vaginal canal upon childbirth. The inner layer of the uterus is composed of an epithelial tissue called the *endometrium*. An increase in the proliferation (division) of endometrial cells can be a sign of *endometrial cancer*, given that cancer is typically marked by high cellular proliferation (Plaxe and Mundt, 2016). Endometrial cancer is currently the fourth most common cancer in women, and it is a strongly established complication of obesity. Endometrial cancer mainly affects women 60 years or older (*post-menopausal*), with a higher prevalence seen in Caucasian women. According to the American Cancer Society, there were more than 60,000 endometrial cancer diagnoses made in 2017, with an estimated fatality count of 10,920 patients in the same year (Key Statistics for Endometrial Cancer? 2017). Multiple studies have determined that there is a positive correlation between an increase in BMI and an increase in a woman's risk for developing endometrial cancer (Schmandt et al, 2011). The factors that are associated with obesity and endometrial cancer involve changes in certain hormone levels, specifically, *estrogen*, a hormone that promotes the growth of the uterine endometrium lining. Although female reproductive organs are abundant normal sources for estrogen, adipose tissue can also produce estrogen, further inducing endometrial growth (Schmandt et al, 2011). Additionally, insulin resistance, which was previously mentioned to have been linked with excess fat tissue and type 2 diabetes, often leads to an increase in insulin in the bloodstream. Elevated insulin levels can indirectly increase proliferation of endometrial cells (Key Statistics for Endometrial Cancer? 2017). Estrogen and insulin play vital roles in promoting natural endometrial growth, but an increase in adipose tissue due to overweight or obesity can negatively alter the rate of growth to the extent that erratic growth can lead to endometrial cancer. Effective therapies that can prevent endometrial cancer caused by obesity include use of oral contraceptives (that regulate estrogen levels), anti-diabetic medications (that lower the cancerous impact of insulin resistance), and behavioral changes (Plaxe and Mundt, 2016; Schmandt et al, 2011).

Other Complications

Besides the medical complications we mentioned, obesity increases your risk of complications if you need surgery for any reason. There are increased risks with getting anesthesia, and with having a complication during or after surgery. Infections, risk of bleeding, and risk of clots after surgery all increase with obesity. Therefore, many doctors require that you be under a certain BMI to even perform a surgery, unless it is an emergency. If you need emergency surgery, there is not much you can do to control this; however, most of us should anticipate that we might need surgery at some point in our life for various reasons, so decreasing your risk beforehand for a better outcome is the goal.

Reproductive Issues

We do not go into details regarding the reproductive organ system, but it is important to know that in men, obesity is linked to erectile dysfunction. In women, it is related to infertility as well as to higher rates of pregnancy complications (including elevated blood pressures and diabetes during pregnancy and Cesarean-sections). Babies of obese mothers have higher rates of health problems during and after birth. Knowing this will give you the power of foresight and make weight loss a central part of your pre-pregnancy planning. If you are planning on becoming pregnant, it is advised that you have a pre-natal appointment with your obstetrician so that you can discuss ways to improve your pre-pregnancy health, for you and your future baby.

What Problems Arise with Anesthesia in Those with Obesity?

When treating obesity, behavioral changes in diet and exercise are commonly prescribed, as these should be the core of any program to achieve and/or maintain a healthy weight. Bariatric (weight-loss) surgery is becoming an increasingly popular alternative method for promoting weight loss in those with moderate to severe obesity, and it might reverse many co-morbidities of obesity. However, patients with obesity can have challenges when responding to anesthesia. Specifically, the physiological changes associated with obesity (like increased respiratory rate, increased total blood volume for circulation, and increased total body weight) often leads to a need for a higher dosage of anesthetic drugs administered, with concomitant increases in the amount of oxygen and blood that are needed during surgery (Schumann, 2016). For example, those with both obesity and obstructive sleep apnea (OSA) might have breathing problems (*hypoventilation*) during operations. Therefore, the increased sensitivity to long-acting sedatives by those with obesity is another challenge in surgery. Proper (and individualized) planning of the anesthesia (general or local) must be done to prevent the occurrence of any problems linked with anesthesia in those with obesity. If you have obesity and OSA, it is important to make sure that your OSA is well treated prior to general surgery.

Conclusion

We have taken time to explore some of the common co-morbidities of obesity (Table 6-4). Some of the described diseases interact with other chronic diseases to further exacerbate the presentation of obesity. For example, type 2 diabetes can occur with both hypertension and gout, leading to a variety of symptoms and to reduced quality of life. The hallmark therapies consistently suggested to be most effective in decreasing these complications are behavioral changes (eating a high-quality diet, conducting physical activity, having high-quality sleep and duration, and reducing stress levels). If behavioral interventions alone are ineffective, you might need to consider weight-loss medications or surgery to help you achieve a healthy weight and better quality of life.

Table 6-4: Common Obesity-Related Complications by Organ System

Organ System				
Cardiovascular	Hypertension	Coronary Artery Disease	Congestive Heart Failure	
Cerebrovascular disease	Thromboembolic disease (TE)			
Pulmonary	Obstructive sleep apnea	Obesity hypoventilation syndrome		
Endocrine	Diabetes mellitus type 2	Hyperlipidemia	Metabolic syndrome	
Gastrointestinal	Non-alcoholic fatty liver disease	Gastroesophageal reflux disease	Cholelithiasis	
Oncologic	Gynecologic/reproductive cancers	Gastrointestinal tract cancers	Urinary tract cancers	Prostate cancer
Musculoskeletal	Osteoarthritis	Gout		
Reproductive	Erectile dysfunction	Infertility	Pregnancy related complications	
Other	Anesthesia or post-surgical complications			

We hope that this chapter provided you with some background information regarding diseases that are linked to obesity. We also hope that it will motivate you and your family to prevent the medical diseases associated with obesity, or if you already have been diagnosed with any, to improve the state of your health. Remember that you are not alone, and that there and many people who are in need of information, just as yourself, and you are brave for seeking help. We hope you can use the information and resources provided to help lead you and your loved ones to a healthier life.

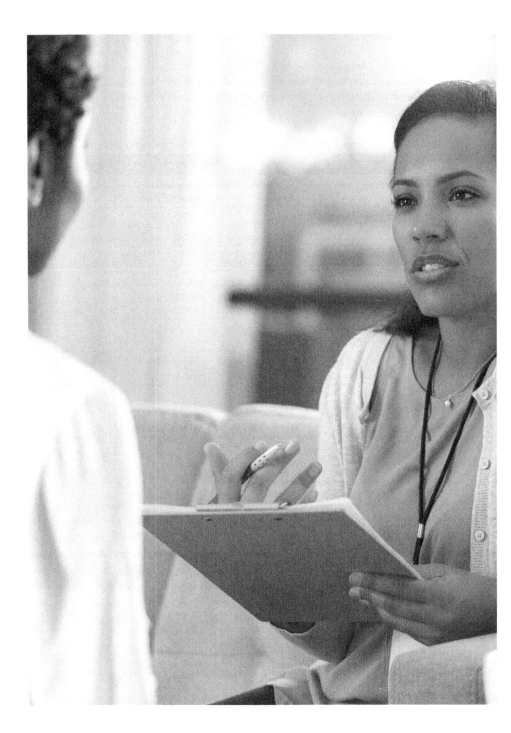

HOW CAN I CALCULATE MY GENETIC RISK FOR OBESITY?

Vibha Singhal, MD

In This Chapter

- Is My Risk for Obesity Inherited?

- How Do I Inherit Genes That Contribute to Obesity?

- How Will I Know Whether My Family Has an Inherited Risk for Obesity?

- Which Types of Obesity Are Linked with an Inherited Risk?

- Should I Discuss Genetic Testing with My Doctor?

- Can I Run into Problems with My Health Insurance Company If It Finds Out That I Am Predisposed to Obesity or Have Obesity?

- Where Can I Get More Information About Being at Risk for Obesity?

Is My Risk for Obesity Inherited?

Obesity occurs for many reasons, some of which are environmental (e.g., the foods we eat, sedentary behaviors, insufficient sleep), whereas others are *genetic* (i.e., the risk we inherit because of being born into a particular family). Your risk for developing obesity increases with the presence of obesity in your parents and family. About 60% to 90% of the risk for obesity is *inherited* (Snyder et al, 2004; Perusse et al, 2005), which means that much of the predisposition to become overweight lies in your *genes*. If one of your parents' struggles with overweight, your risk is two to three times greater than someone who has two lean parents, and it increases about 15-fold if both of your parents suffer from obesity (Whitaker et al, 1997).

Genetic variability can contribute to differences in basic metabolic rate (e.g., how you burn calories), the effects of exercise on weight loss, the utilization of calories, and the response to different kinds of diets on weight-loss efforts. In addition, there are genetic factors that modify your risk of developing complications related to overweight, such as *diabetes, hypertension, heart disease*, and *kidney disease* (Shu et al, 2017).

There are two different kinds of genetic predispositions. With one type, there is an identified defect (*mutation*) in a single gene of your *DNA* that alters the function of that gene. These mutations can be spontaneous (i.e., no defect was present in either parent, but the defective gene can be identified in the person suffering from that disease) or these can be transmitted down generations in a specific manner, such as *autosomal recessive* or *autosomal dominant* (this means that there might be a minor or major contribution to your weight based upon your genes). Less than 1% of obesity is caused by a single gene defect (Reinehr et al, 2007). These single gene defects include certain types of obesity (caused by *proopiomelanocortin* [POMC] *mutations, leptin deficiency, Prader-Willi syndrome, Bardet-Biedl* syndrome) that are inherited in this way. In most instances, the mutated gene is identified by testing. However, because these disorders have a miniscule contribution to the overall prevalence of obesity, they are investigated only when your doctor highly suspects that your obesity has some unique features of these diseases, in addition to obesity.

On the other hand, the more common form of obesity that is caused by caloric excess does not have a single identified and affected gene. This form of obesity, also referred to as *exogenous obesity*, also has a strong genetic predisposition that is attributed to numerous small changes in the whole genome. A recent study suggests that there are about 100 different *loci* (small regions on the DNA) that can be altered to affect the *body mass index* (BMI) (Locke et al, 2015). The contribution of these identified genes to changes in BMI is about 20% (Locke et al, 2015). Unfortunately, there is no commercially available test that looks for these genetic changes. However, there is one gene on chromosome 16 that has gained the most attention: the fat mass and obesity gene, commonly known as the *FTO* gene (Fawcett and Barrosso, 2010). The clear role of the *FTO* gene in causing obesity is still being explored. However, studies suggest that alterations in the *FTO* gene might change the role of some fat cells from using energy to storing energy and slowing down the caloric utilization by *thermogenesis* (Claussnitzer et al, 2015).

How Do I Inherit Genes That Contribute to Obesity?

Genes are the DNA structures that make up *chromosomes*. When conception occurs, half of the genes come from the mother and half come from the father. For the most part, an individual has two copies of a single gene, one from each parent. The physical expression of the gene depends on its dominance (i.e., the more active and stronger the gene, the greater is its expression); sometimes, both genes work equally (called *autosomal recessive*).

There is no one gene that controls the common form of obesity. Scientists have identified many different changes in the DNA that might be associated with the risk of developing obesity, and these small variations are called *single nucleotide polymorphisms* (SNPs). These are small components that alter the function of the gene slightly, but they do not cause a major disruption in its function. These small changes accrue over generations and are then transferred from parents to offspring.

How Will I Know Whether My Family Has an Inherited Risk for Obesity?

If multiple members of your family have struggled with weight for generations, your family likely has the inherited risk of developing obesity. However, it is difficult to know which alterations in the genome are unique to your family. Knowledge of those unique alterations might not have a meaningful impact on your treatment, given that we do not yet know how to reverse these DNA changes.

On the other hand, if you are diagnosed with one of those rare cases of obesity that are caused by single gene defects, certain laboratories can test for this. Tests can also be run on your family members to find out whether they also carry these gene defects.

Which Types of Obesity Are Linked with an Inherited Risk?

Most types of obesity have a genetic predisposition. However, the genetic risk varies with the kind of obesity that you have. As mentioned previously, the rare forms of obesity that have a single identified abnormal gene have a more discrete type of inheritance.

Single gene disorders with obesity as a major trait include the following:

Melanocortin-4 receptor deficiency (MC-4R)

This is the most common cause of obesity associated with a single gene. It can be caused by defects in only one gene (from one parent [*heterozygous*]) or in both genes (from both parents [*homozygous*]).

Leptin deficiency

This is an autosomal recessive condition, in which both genes have a mutation. This typically results in a voracious appetite, high *insulin* levels, *insulin resistance*, and *infertility*.

Leptin receptor deficiency

This is an autosomal recessive condition.

Prohormone convertase-1 deficiency (PCSK1)

This condition involves defects in the production of many hormones. Genetic variability in the gene has been identified.

POMC deficiency

Patients with this condition also have adrenal insufficiency. Genetic changes in both genes have been found.

Syndromes for which obesity is one of the features:

Prader-Willi syndrome

This syndrome is caused by abnormalities in the long arm of chromosome 15. This is the most common syndromic form of obesity. It presents with difficulty feeding at birth and poor muscle tone as a child. There are many behavioral issues, developmental delays, short height, and *hypogonadism*.

Bardet-Biedel syndrome

This is an autosomal recessive condition in which both genes are affected. It is associated with intellectual disability, vision issues, and kidney problems.

Alstrom syndrome

This is a rare autosomal recessive disorder. It usually presents very early in life.

Should I Discuss Genetic Testing with My Doctor?

You should discuss the need for genetic testing with your doctor. However, it is important to realize that the most common kind of obesity does not have a single gene identified as a cause of the obesity. However, the risk of obesity is greater if both parents have obesity than if only one is obese. Although there are many types of changes in the chromosomes, they are now known to contribute a very small fraction to the onset of obesity; knowledge of those changes might not have any direct effect on the treatment of obesity. However, if struggles with weight started in the first few years of life, there might be an indication to look for genes that are known to cause these syndromes. Your doctor will know to look for other symptoms that coexist with obesity, and he or she will order the appropriate test.

Can I Run into Problems with My Health Insurance Company If It Finds Out That I Am Predisposed to Obesity or Have Obesity?

In most cases, obesity will not affect your health insurance status. The Genetic Information Non-discrimination Act (GINA; https://www.genome.gov/27568492/the-genetic-information-nondiscrimination-act-of-2008/) of 2008 prohibits health insurers from discrimination based on knowledge of genetic information. It states that health insurers may not use genetic information to make eligibility, coverage, underwriting, or premium-setting decisions. Typically, if an individual is struggling with weight control, doing the test and getting a positive genetic test does not change any insurance coverage or premiums, as the genetic test just provided an explanation for the problem. For example, a diagnosis of Prader-Willi syndrome would clarify the reasons for obesity and accompanying behavioral issues.

However, genetic testing for *asymptomatic* patients or their relatives can have implications for long-term disability insurance, life insurance, and other medical insurances later in life. In such cases, we counsel families to think about these matters before deciding on testing. This typically applies to a family member whose mother or father has a genetic condition (e.g., *leptin deficiency*), and they want to know whether they might also have it. In that case, if they tested positive, there could be some insurance issues.

Where Can I Get More Information About Being at Risk for Obesity?

The best place to start is with your doctor. He or she can give you information about the likelihood of your genetic risk of obesity. The internet is filled with information, but it is difficult to trust its reliability. There is no risk calculator currently available for the common form of obesity, but if you would like to read more about the genetics of obesity, the following websites can be helpful:

- Pubmed: https://www.ncbi.nlm.nih.gov/pubmed/

- Omim: https://www.omim.org/

- Obesity—medline; https://medlineplus.gov/obesity.html

- The Obesity Society: http://www.obesity.org/resources/facts-about-obesity

- Obesity Action Coalition: http://www.obesityaction.org/educational-resources

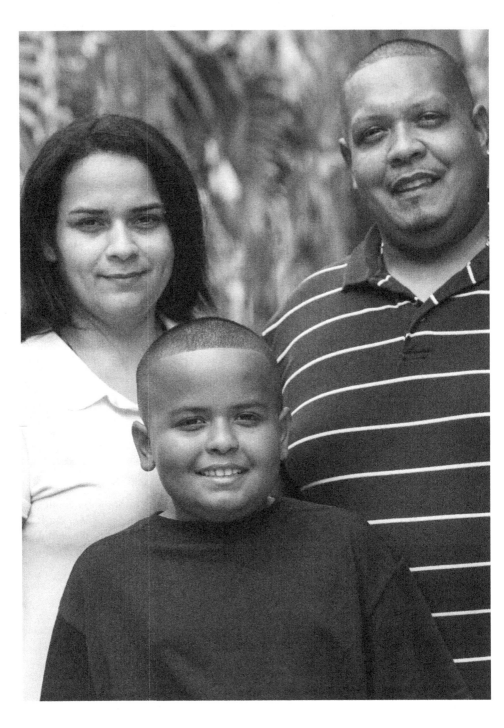

WHAT IMPACT MIGHT MY OBESITY HAVE ON MY FAMILY AND FRIENDS?

Megan Kale Morcomb, LCSW

CHAPTER

In This Chapter

- How Might My Friends and Family Respond to Me If I Have Obesity?

- Is My Family Contributing to My Obesity?

- How Might My Family Change Because of My Obesity?

- What Are Some Indications That My Family Is Not Dealing Well with My Obesity?

- How Might My Own Coping Be Influenced by My Family?

- Is It Wrong for My Family Members to Resent Me and My Obesity?

- What Can My Family Do to Deal More Effectively with My Obesity?

- Are There Support Groups for Family Members of Persons with Obesity?

How Might My Friends and Family Respond to Me If I Have Obesity?

Friends and family will likely have a wide variety of responses to your obesity, which can affect their feelings, thoughts, behaviors, and interactions with you. These responses can be helpful or unhelpful, positive or negative, or even neutral. Some family and friends might respond with mixed feelings about your obesity. Their reactions might be influenced by a range of factors, including the nature of their relationship with you, the severity of your obesity, the impact on your functioning, and their pre-existing thoughts and feelings about obesity. Overall, your family members are more likely to be affected by your obesity than your friends, given that friendships are voluntary and more easily ended when they become strained or unfulfilling, as opposed to family members who are typically more emotionally involved and committed or obligated to maintaining some form of a relationship with you (Carr and Friedman, 2006).

In general, feelings of anxiety, concern, and even fear can play a large role in how your friends, and particularly your family, respond to your obesity. Your family members might worry about your health or the possibility of your developing an associated medical problem, such as *diabetes* or *heart disease*. They might fear that your life will be shortened by an obesity-related illness (NIH, 1998). Family members might worry that they will need to become your caretaker if your obesity is severe or your functioning becomes limited. Others might feel concerned about your mental health being negatively affected, such as having a decline in your self-esteem that results in avoidance and isolation, or the possible development of depression and anxiety (Friedman et al, 2005). Your family might fear that the quality of your life will be impaired and that you might not be able to participate fully in daily activities or in family life due to your obesity. Others might worry about your experiencing stigma, prejudice, and discrimination in the workplace or in society (Carr and Friedman, 2005). They might fear potential job loss or loss of medical insurance coverage. Family and friends might also be concerned about physical barriers or logistical issues about your obesity; for example, not being able to fit into the car comfortably or to find a seat in a public place.

As obesity and related behaviors continue or increase over time, anxiety, fear, and anger can surface among your family members and friends. Because there are many biological, psychological, social, and environmental factors that contribute to the development and continuation of obesity, friends and family members might have difficulty understanding why your obesity has not changed; this leads to frustration. They might also feel discouraged about fluctuations in progress, setbacks, and repeated weight cycling. They might be disappointed and lose trust when promises to change are made but then broken. More than being just frustrated about your obesity, family members and friends are likely to become angry about your unhealthy behaviors that have a negative impact on your lives together

(Carr and Friedman, 2006). For example, family members and friends might be the most upset and resentful about behaviors that disturb your life and their relationships with you, such as compulsive eating, binging or purging, hiding or lying about food, unhealthy dieting, isolating and withdrawing from others, avoiding intimacy, and centering daily activities around food or on weight. There can also be anger regarding money spent on food or obesity-related illnesses. In cases of severe obesity, family members might become angry about having to help with hygiene or self-care. Gradually, these kinds of behaviors can lead to the development of significant anger, resentment, and contempt, as well as damage to and the end of relationships (Carr and Friedman, 2006).

Other responses involve feelings of guilt and shame. Some family members feel responsible for your obesity or feel guilty that they have contributed to your obesity or to your life in general. They might also feel embarrassed, ashamed, or even disgusted because of your obesity (Brownell, 2005). These feelings can lead to efforts to "fix" your obesity, such as controlling or monitoring your food intake, giving excessive advice, belittling or shaming you, or being overly involved. Conversely, others who feel guilty about your obesity might deny that your obesity could be a problem.

Apart from denial about obesity, some family members or friends normalize obesity and do not view it as a problem (Christakis and Fowler, 2007). A large proportion of the population is overweight, and individuals who do not weigh much above the norm might not be seen as having a significant issue. This can also occur in races and ethnic groups in which a heavier body type is considered as more socially acceptable (Carr and Friedman, 2005). Even in groups in which obesity is significantly stigmatized, there can be a sense of camaraderie, normalizing, and rationalizing between obese or otherwise stigmatized individuals, as people tend to choose friends who are like them. Sometimes, these bonds can be threatened when your obesity status changes. In these kinds of relationships, your friends or family members might rationalize their unhelpful behaviors, such as over-eating with you, or attempting to support, comfort or connect with you using food. At times, these individuals overtly or subconsciously thwart your attempts at change. Likewise, feelings of pity can also lead to minimizing or sabotaging behavior.

Family and friends can also respond to your obesity with acceptance and compassion, acknowledging your strengths and enjoying and loving you for who you are. These people might understand the challenges associated with being obese, but they do not define you, your character, or their relationship with you as being based on your weight. However, it is important to understand that even when trying to respond with support and empathy, others might not readily acknowledge your obesity, because they do not want to say the wrong thing and upset you. Even when you are identifying obesity as something you want to change or are identifying personal goals related to developing a healthier lifestyle, family members and friends might minimize the significance of your obesity or the need for an intervention due to their discomfort about hurting your feelings.

Is My Family Contributing to My Obesity?

In thinking about how your family members or family dynamics might be affecting your obesity, it can be helpful to reflect on your current family as well as your family of origin. Both your present and past family systems could be contributing to your obesity.

Dietary habits that you were exposed to as a child can directly affect your current eating behaviors. Perhaps you were raised in a family that did not prepare meals frequently, and you never became confident about learning to cook. Maybe you came from a family that ate a lot of fast food or frozen meals. Growing up, your family might not have been able to afford healthier food options. Your parents might not have been knowledgeable about healthy diets or could have provided you with misinformation about nutrition. Perhaps you were restricted from food as a punishment and bribed or rewarded with food for good behavior. You might have also learned to soothe yourself by eating instead of talking about your feelings or you observed your parents eating when they were upset. These types of scenarios influence what you have internalized about food and eating, thereby affecting your current diet and behaviors (Cruwys et al, 2015).

In addition to reflecting on your past, consider how your current family's habits might be contributing toward your obesity. For example, a spouse might choose to buy or stock up on unhealthy foods that are tempting to over-eat (like chips, candy, and cookies). Children might not want to eat healthier foods or change their diet. Instead of structured mealtimes, family members might eat sporadically or graze throughout the day. Some families can be more sedentary and be "couch potatoes" rather than playing together, going outside, or exercising. Your partner or children's sleeping habits can also affect your weight by causing you to stay up late or not get enough sleep, which increases your risk of obesity (Anderson, 2012). You might also feel unable to fit in grocery shopping and time to cook healthy meals on top of your family and work responsibilities. For many, childcare can be overwhelming and time consuming, particularly for mothers, such that parents do not prioritize taking care of themselves, eating healthy meals, or exercising. Overall, these barriers to change by your family members in regard to daily lifestyle choices can contribute to your obesity (Zweickert and Rieger, 2014).

Families often bond over meals; and family gatherings and familial ethnic and cultural practices often center around food; these practices can derail attempts at healthier eating (Zweickert and Rieger, 2014). For example, it is common to munch on snacks during family activities, like a barbecue, or watching sports, television, or movies together. Family gatherings and traditions almost always involve food preparation (like making cookies during the holidays, roasting a turkey on Thanksgiving, or simply going to get ice cream on the weekend). Immigrant families might also connect and teach younger generations about their culture by preparing meals from their homeland and eating together. During family gatherings, there can be an excess of tempting options and limited or no access to healthier choices. In addition, because these events often revolve around eating, it could be considered offensive not to partake, and there can be pressure for you to eat when you're not hungry. Eating or drinking to manage social stress or to deal with underlying tensions among family members can also occur (Exline et al, 2012).

A history of stressful or traumatic life events and unhealthy family dynamics can contribute toward the development or exacerbation of obesity (Carr and Friedman, 2006). Research has established a strong correlation between stressful life events and the development of obesity. For example, a history of childhood trauma such as parental separation and parental death has been linked to obesity later in life (Alciati et al, 2017). Childhood abuse and neglect, including exposure to domestic violence, and particularly sexual abuse, are commonly associated with the development of obesity (Alvarez et al, 2007). A family history of eating disorders, mental illness, alcoholism, and other addictions can also have a negative impact (D'Argenio et al, 2009).

Stressful circumstances, feeling out of control, and experiencing conflict in your family or marriage can contribute to compulsive eating and obesity. For example, tending to a fussy baby or parenting a child with a disability can be stressful and result in overeating. Caring for aging parents or trying to cope with bereavement can be similarly stressful. Having a spouse who is unemployed or having financial stressors can make healthy eating difficult. Marital conflict has also been linked with appetite dysregulation. Unresolved negative feelings between you and your partner or spouse are likely to contribute toward overeating (Jaremka et al, 2016). Conflict, criticism, and blame can be particularly detrimental (Weihs et al, 2002). Having a spouse or a partner with an untreated addiction, mental illness, or an eating disorder will also likely negatively affect you. Moreover, being in an abusive romantic relationship might exacerbate feelings of low self-esteem and perpetuate coping by overeating, further intensifying poor self-image. Having a partner with low self-esteem can also contribute toward your obesity by enabling or sabotaging behaviors, such as your partner supplying unhealthy food, inciting binge eating, or denying the problem; some partners fear that if their loved one loses weight, he or she might leave them (Carr and Friedman, 2006). Others might encourage over-eating so that they can binge eat with you and decrease their guilt. In some situations, obesity itself can become a scapegoat for difficulties in the relationship to avoid acknowledging or taking responsibility for other problems.

Overall, dietary and lifestyle choices, resistance to change, stressors, interpersonal dynamics, unresolved conflict, abuse, trauma, grief, and loss in a family can contribute to obesity. Although you cannot change your past, exploring how it might affect your obesity in the present, often with the help of a professional, can help you uncover complex psychological processes, dysfunctional family dynamics, and even family habits that contribute toward your obesity.

How Might My Family Change Because of My Obesity?

The more your obesity negatively affects you, the more your family might change, and this can affect your ability to function. If you are constantly focused on your weight, your relationships are likely to suffer. For example, you might miss out on quality time with your family due to being unable to participate in activities because you lack the energy or physical ability to play with or keep up with your children or partner. You might have difficulty traveling and miss out on family events due to your size or a decline in your mobility. If your obesity is related to feeling bad about yourself, your response to these feelings might also change your family dynamics. You might push loved ones away or withdraw from your family. If you are experiencing low self-esteem, it might be difficult to stand up for yourself or ignore family problems that need to be addressed. You might also contribute to conflict by not facing your obesity and instead blame or attack family members.

Your obesity can also change your romantic relationships. Decreased quality time spent together can damage your relationship if you are preoccupied with weight loss. Obesity and poor body image might diminish your level of physical affection and sexual intimacy with your partner (Shah, 2009). If your obesity significantly affects your health and daily functioning, your spouse can end up becoming more of a caretaker than a romantic partner. Your relationship can also become strained if your obesity triggers controlling behaviors in your partner, such as attempting to monitor your food intake or your spending on groceries and food. Eventually, feelings of anxiety, anger, resentment, and disappointment related to obesity could lead to heightened conflict and can result in the ending of a marriage and dissolution of a family.

In addition to the possibility of heightened parental conflict, your children's lives might change in other ways because of your obesity. It is difficult to teach healthy lifestyle choices to children if you are modeling unhealthy behaviors; your children are more likely to become obese (Rhee, 2008; Kimbro et al, 2007). You might also be unintentionally teaching maladaptive coping strategies, or impeding their emotional development if you are preoccupied with your weight, have low self-esteem yourself, or soothe or numb your feelings by eating compulsively.

Your family's financial status might also change because of your obesity. You might have difficulty finding or keeping a job due to physical limitations or associated health concerns. Your family might be adversely affected financially by experiencing stigma that surrounds your obesity. Health concerns related to obesity might also significantly change your family by increasing stress linked to caretaking. Your family might accrue expensive medical bills or have difficulty obtaining insurance. At worst, your lifespan can be shortened, forever changing your family.

What Are Some Indications That My Family Is Not Dealing Well with My Obesity?

There can be a perception that you are not hurting anyone but yourself if you are overeating or are obese; however, we know that this might not be the case. It is better to acknowledge the signs that your family is having a difficult time rather than engaging in denial of distress.

The most obvious indications of poor coping are direct expressions of negative emotions (such as anger and resentment) about your obesity. Fighting and arguing about obesity-related behaviors are clear signals; for example, a spouse expressing frustration about avoidance of activities due to his or her weight. Controlling (managing your grocery list, limiting financial means for food, attempting to force you to exercise, or even putting locks on cupboards or the refrigerator) and monitoring behaviors are also strong indicators that your family members or your partner are not dealing well with your obesity.

Somewhat more difficult to detect is an increase in complaints or over-reactions to something minor. For example, a spouse who is complaining about the number of dishes in the sink might be expressing anger about how much you have eaten. Similarly, passive-aggressive comments are often a way to express negative feelings about a situation. Family members might also make shaming or belittling statements to change your behavior because they are dealing poorly with your obesity. Others might express negative feelings by joking about your weight, at your expense, or by indirectly making obesity-related "fat-jokes" (Tucker, 2014).

There can also be more subtle signs that family members are struggling with your obesity. Some feel embarrassed or uncomfortable with your obesity and distance themselves from you. For example, an adolescent might not want to invite a friend over after school because he or she is embarrassed by your obesity. Family members might also avoid discussing your obesity and related problems or avoid being around you. You might find that you and your partner are spending less and less time together. A spouse or partner might avoid physical affection or sexual intimacy.

Even though they might not understand whether a situation is obesity related, children often express sadness or guilt about behaviors they observe in a parent, given that children are more likely to attribute blame to themselves than to a parent. Some children express confusion or seem sad about their obese parent's behavior. For example, a parent might avoid taking their child to the park because of weight-related issues, but the child interprets this as being because of some defect within themselves or feel unloved or abandoned, not comprehending the real reason. In addition, because of stress on the family system, some children act out or misbehave, whereas others attempt to be perfect. Because your children think concretely and have less capacity for emotional regulation than adults, you might need to observe carefully for indications that your children are not handling your obesity well, because it might not be as clear as with your adult family members.

How Might My Own Coping Be Influenced by My Family?

Everyone uses coping strategies to manage feelings and to deal with problems. Some of these methods are learned from our families and others we glean from later-life experience. Regarding obesity, it can be helpful to reflect on how over-eating might have become a maladaptive coping strategy and whether you and your family members are coping well with emotions or life stressors (Weihs et al, 2002). In some families, eating can become a primary method of coping with unexpressed negative feelings. Family members sometimes learn that eating makes them feel better or distracts them from their emotions. Some people eat to cope with feelings of sadness, loneliness, boredom, emptiness, anxiety, disappointment, anger, guilt, and shame. In particular, anger is often an uncomfortable emotion for many families, and it can result in over-eating. Others might eat to re-establish a feeling of control in a chaotic family environment or when they feel helpless and cannot alter their circumstances. Some people eat to cope with the belief that they are not good enough or are unloved (Holland et al, 2012). Unfortunately, feeling stigmatized by one's family because of obesity has been associated with negative coping strategies, such as eating more, avoiding, and ignoring the situation (Puhl et al, 2006).

Being obese can also become a coping strategy for some who have experienced trauma. These individuals can use obesity as a way of coping with vulnerability because they feel safer and better able to protect themselves when their bodies are larger. Others use obesity as a deterrent against unwanted attention.

If you suspect that you or your family members are not coping well or are using unhealthy strategies for dealing with intense emotions and stress, it can help to seek professional support. It is unlikely that you will be able to lose weight and keep it off over the long term if there are unaddressed issues and ineffective coping skills that are affecting your obesity rather than just eating a poor diet or lacking exercise (Alvarez et al, 2007).

Is It Wrong for My Family Members to Resent Me and My Obesity?

As human beings, we would all like to be loved and accepted unconditionally by our families, and it can be extremely challenging to feel resented for having obesity. However, negative feelings about your obesity can develop slowly among your family members; and although some reactions might be unhelpful, or downright hurtful, your family members are entitled to their feelings, just as you can have your feelings. If you believe your family members resent your obesity, try to consider their point of view and the reasons that might be causing them to feel this way.

If your family members' lives are being negatively affected by your obesity, their resentment can be understandable. For example, resentment might be a reasonable response if your eating or obesity result in isolation and alienation from your loved ones. Self-destructive, obsessive, and compulsive behaviors are also likely to trigger anger from your family. Lying about as well as spending excessive amounts of money on food or weight-loss products can also lead to similar reactions. Other eating-disordered behaviors such as binging and purging are also understandably distressing to family members (Carr and Friedman, 2006).

In contrast, resentment can be the result of a deeper issue in a relationship that might be obscured because of a focus on obesity. Because obesity is so visible and cannot be concealed, it can become a scapegoat for other problems in a relationship; other issues can be overlooked because the obesity is more apparent. For example, if one spouse has compulsive over-eating and the other has irritability related to anxiety, the obesity can be the more obvious of the two, although both problems are likely to negatively affect the marriage.

Overall, relationships are quite complicated and are affected by a variety of factors. If you feel like a partner or family member is resentful of you apart from your obesity, it can be important for you and maybe even for that individual to seek help, especially if you want to preserve or to improve the relationship. Working with a professional can help you process hurt feelings and establish realistic expectations. And, talking with someone who has an outsider's perspective can help you discern your responsibility for the situation without taking on excessive blame. In time, relationships can heal when there is acknowledgment of how others have been negatively affected. However, it is important to understand that change is still possible, even if you do not ever get the kind of support you want from your family.

What Can My Family Do to Deal More Effectively with My Obesity?

One of the most important things for family members to do is to take responsibility for their feelings, thoughts, and behaviors and to evaluate their involvement and personal ways of coping. Obesity is not something that family members can cure or solve for a loved one. Ideally, family members need to learn how to set boundaries and to make choices so as not to suffer the consequences of someone else's condition and choices. Ultimately, it is the responsibility of the person with obesity to seek health in ways that work. For family members, taking ownership and setting boundaries could mean stopping controlling behaviors or trying to fix the obese person. It could be expressing thoughts and emotions about the situation, gently but honestly, rather than attacking, being passive-aggressive, or avoiding the topic. It might include identifying and stopping enabling or sabotaging behaviors. Trying to listen and providing acceptance might be better than giving advice.

Accepting that obesity is a disease with multiple and complex causes and separating the person and their character from the disease, can be a helpful way to reframe the situation. Families can take comfort in the fact that they can still love and be supportive without having to like or approve of their obesity or related behaviors. Other ways to manage more effectively involve identifying and addressing unhelpful thoughts, such as black-or-white and all-or-nothing thinking. Recognizing cognitive distortions (such as the false belief that if they loved me, they would not over-eat or be obese) is also important. Other ways family members can more effectively cope is by focusing on strengths and successes rather than on failures.

Personal change is not linear, and there will be ups and downs along the way; obesity is not something that is alleviated overnight and might present a life-long struggle. It is imperative for families to support mental and physical health and relationship building, as opposed to just weight loss by the person with obesity. Family members will fare better by making a commitment to their emotional and physical well-being, having compassion, and setting appropriate boundaries. If these objectives seem overwhelming, and they can be, seek help from a professional or a support group to facilitate change and obtain additional support.

Are There Support Groups for Family Members of Persons with Obesity?

Obtaining outside support can be particularly helpful for both the obese person as well as their family members, and there are multiple options available, although access can vary depending on where you live. In general, support groups are led by peers or group members, whereas therapy groups are led by clinicians or other professionals. In addition, individual, couples, or family therapy can be beneficial (Weihs et al, 2002). Individual therapy can be useful for the person with obesity as well as for family members to process and explore their feelings, whereas couples or family therapy will address problems and unhelpful family dynamics together. These options have different benefits and can be complementary to one another. Initially, you might try a few different groups or providers to find the best fit for you and your family.

If you are unsure about the options available in your area, start by asking a *primary-care physician, endocrinologist, bariatric surgeon, psychiatrist*, or other physician specialist for a referral suggestions. *Social workers*, marriage and *family therapists*, and licensed professional counselors might also be able to direct you to local clinicians or support groups that specialize in obesity or eating disorders. *Nutritionists* and *dietitians* can also be excellent referral sources. In addition, there are on-line resources that have national directories that can help you and your family members locate appropriate support, such as the *National Eating Disorder Association* (NEDA) (www.nationaleatingdisorders.org) and the *National Association of Anorexia Nervosa and Associated Disorders* (ANAD) (www.anad.org).

Overeaters Anonymous (OA) (www.oa.org) is a free member-led organization with support groups across the country. *Al-Anon* and *Alateen* (www.al-anon.alateen.org) provide specific support for adult and adolescent family members of a person with addiction. Although these latter two groups are generally considered to be for family members of alcoholics, they can still be quite useful for family members of an obese person because many of the same family dynamics apply. Lastly, although you might not consider obesity to be an eating disorder, do not rule out eating-disordered options prematurely, as eating-disordered behaviors encompass a wide variety of behaviors, including those that are related to obesity.

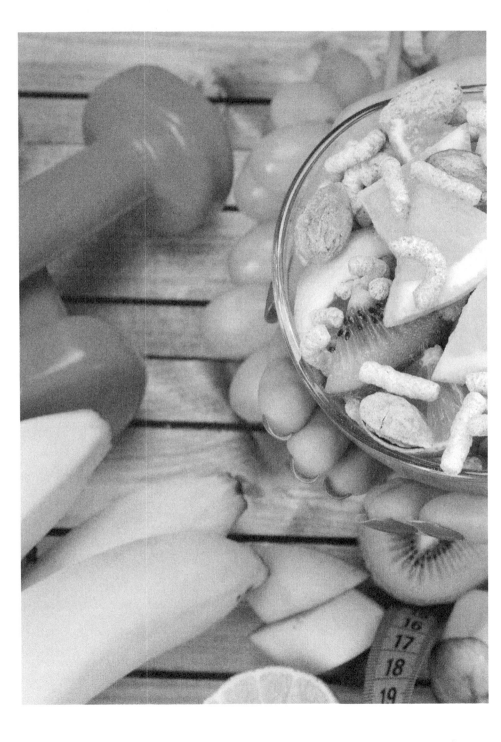

WHAT LIFESTYLE CHANGES CAN I MAKE TO ADDRESS MY OBESITY?

Kim George, MS, RD, LD

CHAPTER

In This Chapter

- In General, How Can Obesity Affect My Lifestyle?

- Should I Go on a Diet?

- Should I Change How I Am Eating?

- Are There Certain Foods That I Should Avoid to Lose Weight?

- Do I Need to Drink 8 Cups of Water Daily?

- What Is Emotional Eating?

- Is It Safe to Exercise While I Have Excess Weight?

- How Often Should I Exercise?

- What Kind of Exercise Should I Do?

- Should I Attempt to Stop Drinking Alcohol or Smoking Cigarettes?

In General, How Can Obesity Affect My Lifestyle?

Lifestyle modification, also referred to as *behavioral weight control*, includes three primary components: diet, exercise, and behavioral therapy.

Everyday activities that many people take for granted are affected by excessive weight. If you struggle with obesity you are probably familiar with its many physical and emotional consequences. Extra body weight makes getting up from a chair or walking more difficult. You might find yourself struggling to catch your breath after walking to a store or while preparing dinner. You might also become tired more easily, and you are at an increased risk for a host of diseases and illnesses. Medical conditions (e.g., *heart disease, stroke, high blood pressure, diabetes, joint pain, respiratory problems, gout, gallstones*) are all worsened by having extra body fat. See Chapter 6 for more information regarding the medical consequences of obesity.

Although your health is jeopardized by having excess weight, many people who need medical attention avoid seeking help or delay making medical appointments due to their fear of being stigmatized because of their excess weight. A dear family friend of mine had rescheduled her yearly physical multiple times for fear that the nurse who weighed her would comment on her weight when she was on the scale. She dreaded going to her appointment. Together, we were able to strategize about how to inform the nurse before being weighed that her weight was a sensitive issue for her. The appointment still caused her anxiety, but she felt better advocating for herself. Many people recognize that obesity can be a target of prejudice and that learning more about stigma can be challenging.

I also worked with someone who had struggled with *anorexia nervosa* as a teenager. As she worked toward recovery and restored her body weight, she continued to struggle with her relationship with food. Later, she became obese as an adult. She decided to write about weight stigma in college and read article after article on weight-biased medical professionals and those in the general public. As she was nearing the end of her research paper she found herself struggling more with her body image and her mental health. *Obesity* plays a significant role in our mental and emotional health. Anxiety, depression, and fear can be problematic and affect our self-esteem. More about weight stigma is presented in Chapter 16. Chapter 2 explains more about depression and moods that are related to obesity. In sum, obesity interferes with all aspects of life.

Should I Go on a Diet?

Information about diets seems to be everywhere (e.g., in the tabloids at the checkout counters [detailing the latest diet of a movie star], talking to colleagues about their newest weight-loss trick, or talking to your uncle about the same 15 pounds he has been losing at Christmas for who knows how many years). Each year, millions of people make a New Year's resolution to lose weight. As a registered dietitian, I'm often asked for my opinion on the best method for losing weight and about how to lose fat and weight quickly. Keep in mind that being obese is a health risk. If you decide to change your eating habits you should focus on making health improvements rather than on decreasing your weight. Weight loss is a billion-dollar industry. If there were one quick, easy, and effective method, there wouldn't be so many different diets; we would all be in a desirable weight range. At the end of the day, weight loss is achieved when our bodies use more energy (calories) than we consume. Our society has made it easy to eat more and to move less. We can pay a mere 50 cents more at a movie theater to get unlimited free refills on our soda and we can use moving walkways in the airport instead of walking.

There is no quick and easy solution for losing weight. Weight loss takes time and commitment. Maintaining weight loss takes even more effort. Losing weight just to lose weight might not be motivation enough to make and maintain lifestyle changes. You should question your motivation to lose weight. Do you want to look good at your sister's wedding? Do you want to decrease your *cholesterol* level and avoid taking another medication?

My advice for a diet—or, better yet, for a lifestyle change—is to identify small, measurable goals toward which you are willing to work. Identify SMART goals: Specific, Measurable, Attainable, Realistic, and Time-bound goals. Identify a clear goal (Specific) that you are able to refer to and ask yourself if you have achieved it (Measurable). Make a goal achievable (Attainable and Realistic) and give yourself a time frame (Time-bound). Regularly evaluate your goals. If you have achieved your goal, how can you maintain your new habits? If you did not achieve your goal, can you break the goal down into a smaller goal or decide whether you need to make a new goal toward which you are ready to work.

For example: Henry, a man who had gained 10 pounds over the past year saw his cholesterol increase to 250 mg/dL. He was prescribed several different medications, and he hated the thought of adding yet another pill to his health regimen. For years, he had wanted to lose weight and started multiple diets but had difficulty continuing with them. When he saw his cholesterol level rise, he wanted to make changes in his nutrition and exercise schedule before deciding to take a new medication. We discussed the *plate method* along with the benefits of exercise and increasing his fiber intake. Henry was attentive and engaged throughout the hour-long nutrition sessions. At the goal-setting point of our session, he identified three goals: losing weight, decreasing his cholesterol level, and eating healthy. Together, we broke down each goal into SMART goals. We noted that Henry typically ate breakfast, worked through lunch, and then visited the vending machine in the late afternoon when he got really hungry. Then, he ate a balanced dinner each night that he made with his partner. Instead of focusing on weight loss, we agreed on more immediate goals (i.e., he would bring lunch from home each day and take a brief break to eat, he would reduce his visits to the vending machine every afternoon). These changes would help him keep from getting too hungry during the afternoon and would assist him in making healthier choices. Although it would be difficult to see whether his cholesterol level had decreased in a few weeks, Henry thought that he was probably not consuming at least

25 grams of fiber each day. He would move his focus from decreasing his cholesterol intake to increasing his fiber intake. He could eat either two slices of whole-grain bread or one cup of cooked oatmeal in the morning. We determined that his goal of eating healthy should be broken down into a more achievable goal. He would follow the plate method at dinner by eating half a plate of vegetables, a fourth of a plate of a starch, and a fourth of a plate of a lean protein. We reviewed his goals during our follow-up session two weeks later. He found that he enjoyed eating his whole grains at breakfast, and he believed that using the plate method at dinner was helpful. Bringing his lunch to work was more difficult because he frequently forgot to bring something from home. This provided us with an opportunity to further break this goal into component parts. We strategized about lunch options. He had already identified that he would benefit from increasing his fiber intake; lunch provided an opportunity to add a fruit serving. When we discussed his favorite fruits, Henry said that his partner had agreed to purchase oranges and apples at the grocery store this week and that he would keep them at his desk at work. He needed a meal that did not require warming and we identified that he would either bring in a sandwich on whole-grain bread (e.g., a salad with chicken and beans, or a wrap) and he would pack his lunch the night before going to work. Every other week Henry would review his goals to identify which ones were working for him and which needed tweaking. At a 6-month follow-up appointment, his cholesterol level was rechecked, and it had decreased to 200 mg/dL. His physician agreed that prescribing additional medications to decrease his cholesterol was not needed.

Should I Change How I Am Eating?

Following a diet can be challenging. Many people want to eat healthily but do not always achieve their goal. One year, our wellness coordinator and I organized a *Fruit and Vegetable Challenge Month* at work. Employees were provided with handouts that we developed; each week, these new goals were to increase the variety of foods eaten and their general intake. I thought that this challenge would be a "no brainer." I'm a registered dietitian, I eat healthily. During the first week, I did amazingly well and I enjoyed eating two fruits daily. As we reached week three, I recognized that eating an adequate amount of fruits and vegetables was easier said than done. I grew tired of eating carrots and hummus as my afternoon snack. Moreover, having a banana for my evening snack was proving to be boring. Where was my variety? My weekend intake record revealed that I rarely ate fruit even though I ate it regularly during the week. My weekends were filled with activities and I was on the go most of the time. At work, I ate at a beautiful fruit bar in the cafeteria and eating fruit there was easy to do. People often think about what they are eating and drinking, but they are often eating and drinking much differently than they had intended. Keeping a weekly log of my vegetable and fruit intake helped me to identify my habits and areas where I could make improvements. If you are uncertain whether you need to make nutritional changes, keep a food log; it can be an easy way for you to guide your eating patterns. I encouraged others to keep a log for 3 to 7 days of everything they ate and drank. It is also helpful to incorporate days off and weekends into your food log because those days have eating patterns that can look very different from those on weekdays. People often forget how many times they dip into a co-worker's candy dish or how many sweetened beverages they consume. A food log reveals our habits; when we are honest with ourselves about what we eat and drink, it can be a real eye-opener. After you establish your typical intake, take a moment to detect patterns. Are you eating on a schedule? Do you tend to skip meals? Do you eat when you are bored, or do you like to get second helpings when there is free food? Creating a food log is a great way to help you identify changes in your diet.

Tactics for eating well involve eating on a schedule, listening to your body (e.g., feelings of hunger and fullness) and enjoying a variety of foods. Try aiming to eat every 3 to 4 hours around the same times each day. Our bodies love being on a schedule. Eating consistently helps us achieve stable blood sugar levels and helps our metabolism (e.g., eating six small meals a day, or three meals a day with several snacks). Meals typically contain larger portions than snacks. Snacks enable us to meet the food group recommendations that you are not eating at regular meals. The plate method is a visual method of organized eating. You can visit choosemyplate.gov to understand more about creating portions and following recommendations from each food group. The plate method encourages you to fill half of your plate with fruits and vegetables; a quarter of your plate having lean proteins, and a quarter of your plate filled with starchy foods. After you have incorporated dairy and sparingly added oils or fats, you will have gathered all of your food groups. Recommended portion sizes vary frequently from what most people eat in one meal.

I had a client, Caroline, who wanted to become pregnant but was having difficulties conceiving due to *polycystic ovarian syndrome*. Her physician recommended that she make lifestyle changes to improve her chances of becoming more fertile. Caroline and I met to achieve balanced eating to improve her blood sugars. I educated her on the plate method and she was surprised by my recommendation to eat six servings of starches daily. She explained that she was only eating three servings daily and was reluctant to increase her intake. We reviewed her typical day and she explained that she usually ate a bagel with cream cheese early in the morning as she left for work. For lunch she ate a turkey and cheese sandwich, potato chips, and a soda (that she packed at home). Around 2:30 p.m. she would meet her co-worker for a coffee break and eat a yogurt with granola with a large vanilla latte. Dinner typically consisted of chicken or fish with a large salad. Before bed, she and her husband ate ice cream together. Together, we discovered her bagel was equivalent to four starches, her lunch provided another four starches (due to the chips and the two slices of bread) and her afternoon snack contained one starch (the granola), totaling nine starches. We noticed that her dinner was light and it left her hungry after an hour or so, when she ate the equivalent of three servings of ice cream. Caroline identified that she could switch her bagel to two slices of whole-grain bread with peanut butter and a banana, pack a wrap with a small tortilla (with turkey and cheese), a pear, and a sparkling water, and she could continue to eat her yogurt and granola as her snack and switch to water from the vanilla latte. She and her husband decided to add rice, potatoes, or corn to their dinner to promote fullness and decrease their ice cream servings to two scoops and use a smaller bowl. Caroline felt these goals were simple yet powerful exchanges. Within the next 6 months her menstrual cycles became more regular and she was delighted to share that she was pregnant.

Listening to our bodies for feelings of hunger and fullness sounds easy, but it can prove to be quite difficult. Do you know when you begin to feel hungry? Can you pinpoint during a meal when you are reaching satisfaction? Many people eat so quickly that they do not take the time to assess how their body is feeling before, during, and after a meal. As discussed earlier, eating every 3 to 4 hours is key to achieving balanced eating. Check in with your body and make sure that you start to eat a meal or snack before you are ravenous. The ability to achieve balanced eating goes out the window when we are hungry. As you begin to eat notice the texture, taste, and smell of your food. Take time to enjoy the flavors. Assess your fullness throughout the eating episode. Roughly 5 to 7 minutes into a meal you should ask yourself if you are eating for hunger or because there is still food on your plate. Try to feel the sensation of fullness arriving. Put your fork down throughout the meal and take time to chew and to drink your beverage. Continue to eat until you are satisfied, and you will be satisfied for the next 3 to 4 hours. After you eat, notice how you feel. If you feel full after a meal remember what that experience feels like so that you can stop eating sooner during the next meal. If you are hungry an hour after a meal, you might not have eaten enough at the meal or snack. Respect your hunger and your fullness; with practice, you will be better at eating for your bodies' energy needs. Use the Hunger/Fullness Scale (see Table 9-1) to help you identify where you are with your hunger before, during, and after a meal.

Table 9-1: Hunger/Fullness Scale

1	Empty, starving, weak, shaky, difficulty concentrating
2	Irritable, cranky, decreased energy, "hangry"
3	Time to eat, hungry
4	Less hungry, thinking more about food
5	Neutral
6	Almost satisfied but not quite there
7	Satisfied and likely to be satisfied for 3 to 4 hours
8	Feeling too full, a few bites too many
9	Uncomfortable, bloated
10	Feeling sick from fullness, "Thanksgiving Day" fullness

Just as eating on a schedule and respecting your hunger and fullness are essential for balanced eating, so too is eating a variety of foods. Each food group provides your body with key nutrients. Within each food group, the different colors and types of foods provide you with a variety of nutrient profiles. Try to eat foods that have different colors within the fruit and vegetable groups. Taste the rainbow! Each color provides you with a different *anti-oxidant*. If you eat the same foods each day you are eating the same nutrients, which also means that you are missing the same nutrients each day. Eating a variety of foods helps to keep meals interesting.

Are There Certain Foods That I Should Avoid to Lose Weight?

There are no good or bad foods. Most people have difficulty with eating appropriate portions. A well-balanced eating plan should not encourage you to avoid either certain foods or entire food groups without medical necessity. There are no perfect foods nor is one food superior to another. Kale is a great food but it does not contain all the nutrients that your body requires. Your body deserves to eat a variety of foods from each food group to meet its nutritional needs. Each food group provides your body with different macro and micro nutrients. Due to the diverse nature of nutrients provided by each group you need to select different portions from each group.

Several sources of information provide their own unique recommendations so that you can meet your energy requirements. MyPlate Daily Checklist, which you can find on choosemyplate.gov, provides examples of food group recommendations for various calorie allowances. A person's food plan is personalized (based on age, gender, height, weight, and physical activity level). The website has a MyPlate Checklist Calculator to help you determine calorie estimates. The calculator provides you with a food pattern to maintain your current weight and another food pattern to help you promote weight loss. These food patterns are a great place to begin. Each pattern provides recommendations with portion sizes from each food group. You might find that more support is necessary to assist you with weight loss. Losing weight and maintaining weight loss is difficult. *Registered dietitians* are nutrition experts who can guide you to balanced and appropriate food decisions. Registered dietitians are trained in best practices and evidence-based choices.

I call foods that do not easily fit into a food group "fun foods" (such as cookies, cakes, pies, candy, or even fried foods). Many people elect to restrict these foods when they decide that they are going to eat better. All food is allowed in moderation. If you tell yourself you cannot have a cookie, what do you often find yourself craving? A cookie! This does not mean that you should eat cookies to your heart's content. Remember, we need to honor our hunger and our fullness. Identify what "moderation of fun foods" looks like to you. I love fun foods, and I try to aim for one portion daily, although my husband aims to eat fun foods three times a week.

I had a client, Raymond, who wanted to change his eating habits, and he was encouraged to do so by his physician. Raymond had tried to lose weight numerous times, but he frequently became frustrated when he could not eat perfectly. He enjoyed socializing and found that when he was trying to lose weight, his friends frequently wanted to go out for ice cream or go to the movies (where he had difficulty saying "no" to popcorn). When he was trying to eat healthier, he either avoided going to the movies to eat well or he threw caution to the wind and ate whatever he wanted. He had difficulty balancing his social life with sensible eating. As we discussed, moderation and not visualizing healthy eating are not all-or-nothing. Raymond realized that he could have the best of both worlds. He could permit himself to enjoy fun foods three times a week. He could enjoy popcorn at the movies by choosing a small bag with light butter and he could drink water instead of soda. When his friends decided to go out for ice cream he "passed" on the banana split and enjoyed a medium size ice cream portion, instead. Raymond simply had to choose when he was going to enjoy his fun foods. At times, this meant deciding to have the ice cream on Thursday and to substitute broccoli for onion rings on Friday. Raymond learned to enjoy his fun foods in moderation and he no longer felt the need to "throw in the towel" on his balanced eating.

Do I Need to Drink 8 Cups of Water Daily?

The amount of fluid you need depends on your medical conditions, body weight, and physical activity. A quick way to calculate your fluid requirement is to divide your weight in pounds by two, to equal how many ounces of fluid you require daily. For example, if you weigh 250 pounds: 250/2 = 125 ounces or 15.6 cups of water. You get fluid not only from what you drink but also from the foods you eat. Drinking an adequate amount of fluid is necessary for your overall health. Fluids assist in breaking down food, move nutrients throughout your body, regulate body temperature, and are essential for all cells to function. Our thirst mechanism can be difficult to identify and many people think that they are hungry when they are actually thirsty. If you want a quick method to determine whether you are well hydrated, inspect your urine and aim for the color of light lemonade. Be mindful to limit sweetened beverages, they add calories quickly.

What Is Emotional Eating?

Emotional eating is using food to manage your emotions (i.e., to self-soothe). You might not even recognize when you are engaging in emotional eating. Happiness, sadness, boredom, excitement, loneliness, stress, anger, regret, and fear are all emotions that can lead to eating when you are not hungry. Many well-planned diets have been hijacked by emotional eating. I encourage my clients to "hit the pause button" when eating outside of their normal eating times. Pause, and ask yourself whether you are hungry or merely eating to relieve emotions. How do you feel? If you have identified that you are eating to modify an emotion, the next step is to face the emotion head on. I had a client, Sarah, who struggled with emotional eating. She was an accountant who noticed that she always gained weight around tax season; over the years the weight had piled on. She noticed that on the evenings when she worked late, she felt drained after returning home. She frequently reached for her favorite cookies and a glass of cold milk. This was her method of treating herself after a long day at the office. Although she enjoyed the milk and cookies, she recognized that she was not truly hungry and she was using the snack to self-soothe. Sarah was encouraged to identify alternative strategies for relaxing instead of eating. She discovered that she enjoyed watching a few minutes of funny YouTube videos. Sarah noticed that she felt better, laughed, and her mood lifted after seeing silly cats dancing. It is useful to have a variety of alternative self-soothing options (e.g., coloring, listening to music, taking a bath or shower, reading, knitting, working on a puzzle, calling a friend, gardening, taking a walk, meditating). You might make a list of what you enjoy and practice using the list when you are finding yourself eating in the absence of hunger. Alternative coping skills are a great way to self-soothe, but keep in mind that it is important to address your emotions. Avoiding emotions will not make them disappear. We need to allow ourselves to experience our emotions.

Is It Safe to Exercise While I Have Excess Weight?

Exercise provides you with physical and emotional benefits. Physical activity decreases the risk of premature death, heart problems, stroke, type 2 diabetes, certain cancers, falls, and depression. Exercise aids in bone health, cardiorespiratory and muscular health, concentration, and it provides you with a feeling of mastery. Prior to making radical changes it is a good idea to discuss with your medical team whether exercise is safe and appropriate for you. Your medical team will help you determine your appropriate activity level. After you are cleared to begin an exercise program, begin slowly and gradually increase the intensity level. I had a client, John, who was excited about making lifestyle changes, and he began exercising. He joined a local gym and began working out. He excelled in exercising with others and he enjoyed the comradery, competition, and opportunity to create new friendships. The trainer at the gym encouraged John to listen to his body and take a rest, if needed, during the workouts. John was enjoying the class during the first week and finding himself in competition with others in the room. However, he developed muscle pain, felt tired, and noticed that his urine had turned dark brown. He made a medical appointment to discuss his symptoms. His doctor discovered that one of his blood tests, creatine kinase, was elevated and he was diagnosed with rhabdomyolysis (a condition associated with muscle breakdown). Thankfully, John received treatment in a timely fashion and he recovered with administration of fluids; subsequently, he was able to slowly increase his physical activity again. This time he followed the trainer's advice and rested during workouts. It is important not to push yourself too hard. You want to incorporate exercise into your lifestyle and make it something that you enjoy rather than dread.

How Often Should I Exercise?

There are many different sets of recommendations for exercise. Table 9-2 provides a summary of exercise regimens.

Table 9-2: Recommendations for Exercise According to Leading Organizations

American Heart Association (AHA) http://www.heart.org/HEARTORG/ HealthyLiving/PhysicalActivity/FitnessBasics/ American-Heart-Association-Recommendations-for-Physical-Activity-in-Adults_UCM_307976_ Article.jsp#.WRUMgPnyuM8	For overall cardiovascular health: • At least 30 minutes of moderate-intensity aerobic activity at least 5 days each week for a total of 150 minutes per week OR • At least 25 minutes of vigorous aerobic activity at least 3 days per week for a total of 75 minutes per week; or a combination of moderate- and vigorous-intensity aerobic activity AND • Moderate- to high-intensity muscle-strengthening activity at least 2 days per week to attain additional health benefits. For lowering blood pressure and cholesterol levels: • An average of 40 minutes of moderate- to vigorous-intensity aerobic activity three or four times each week
National Heart, Lung, and Blood Institute https://www.nhlbi.nih.gov/health/health-topics/ topics/phys/recommend	Adults: • People obtain health benefits from as little as 60 minutes of moderate-intensity aerobic activity each week. • For major health benefits, one should do at least 150 minutes of moderate-intensity aerobic activity or 75 minutes of vigorous-intensity aerobic activity each week. Another option is to do a combination of the two. A general rule is that 2 minutes of moderate-intensity activity is equivalent to 1 minute of vigorous-intensity activity. • For even more health benefits, do 300 minutes of moderate-intensity aerobic activity or 150 minutes of vigorous-intensity activity per week (or a combination of the two). The more active you are, the more benefits you will receive.

National Heart, Lung, and Blood Institute https://www.nhlbi.nih.gov/health/health-topics/topics/phys/recommend *(continued)*	• When performing aerobic activity, do it for at least 10 minutes at a time. Spread the activity throughout the week. Muscle-strengthening activities that are of moderate or vigorous intensity should be included 2 or more days per week. These activities should work on all of the major muscle groups (legs, hips, back, chest, abdomen, shoulders, and arms). Examples include lifting weights, working with resistance bands, and doing sit-ups and push-ups, yoga, and heavy gardening.
	Adults aged 65 or older:
	• Older adults should be physically active. Older adults who do any amount of physical activity will gain some health benefits.
	• Older adults should be active. Older adults who do any amount of physical activity gain health benefits.
	• If you can't do 150 minutes of activity each week, be as physically active as your abilities and condition will allow.
World Health Organization http://www.who.int/dietphysicalactivity/factsheet_adults/en/	• Adults aged 18–64 years should do at least 150 minutes of moderate-intensity aerobic activity throughout the week or do at least 75 minutes of vigorous-intensity aerobic activity throughout the week or an equivalent combination of moderate- and vigorous-intensity activity.
	• Aerobic activity should be performed in blocks of at least 10 minutes.
	• For additional health benefits, adults should increase their moderate-intensity aerobic physical activity to 300 minutes per week, or engage in 150 minutes of vigorous-intensity aerobic activity per week, or an equivalent combination of moderate- and vigorous-intensity activity.
	• Muscle-strengthening activities should involve major muscle groups on 2 or more days per week.

continued

Center for Disease Control and Prevention https://www.cdc.gov/physicalactivity/basics/adults/index.htm	• One should engage in 150 minutes of moderate-intensity aerobic activity and muscle strengthening activities on 2 or more days each week that works on all major muscle groups Or • 75 minutes of vigorous-intensity aerobic activity and muscle strengthening activities on 2 or more days each week that work all muscle groups Or • An equivalent mix of moderate and vigorous-intensity aerobic activity and muscle-strengthening activities on 2 or more days that work all major muscle groups
American College of Sports Medicine http://www.acsm.org/about-acsm/media-room/news-releases/2011/08/01/acsm-issues-new-recommendations-on-quantity-and-quality-of-exercise	Cardiorespiratory exercise: • Adults should get at least 150 minutes of moderate-intensity exercise per week. • Exercise recommendations can be met through 30 to 60 minutes of moderate-intensity exercise (5 days per week) or 20 to 60 minutes of vigorous-intensity exercise (3 days per week). • One continuous session and multiple shorter sessions (of at least 10 minutes) are both acceptable to accumulate the desired amount of exercise. • Gradual progression of exercise time, frequency, and intensity is recommended for best adherence and the lowest risk of injury. • People unable to meet these minimums can still benefit from enjoying some activity. Resistance exercise: • Adults should train each major muscle group 2 or 3 days per week using a variety of exercises and equipment. • Very light or light intensity is best for older persons or previously sedentary adults starting exercise. • Two to four sets of each exercise will help adults improve their strength and power.

American College of Sports Medicine http://www.acsm.org/about-acsm/media-room/ news-releases/2011/08/01/acsm-issues-new- recommendations-on-quantity-and-quality- of-exercise *(continued)*	• For each exercise, 8 to 12 repetitions improve strength and power, 10 to 15 repetitions improve strength in middle-age and older persons starting exercise, and 15 to 20 repetitions improve muscular endurance. • Adults should wait at least 48 hours between resistance-training sessions. Flexibility exercise: • Adults should do flexibility exercises at least 2 or 3 days per week to improve their range of motion. • Each stretch should be held for 10 to 30 seconds to the point of tightness or slight discomfort. • Each stretch should be repeated two to four times, accumulating 60 seconds/stretch. • Static, dynamic, ballistic, and PNF stretches are all effective. • Flexibility exercises are most effective when muscles are warm. Try light aerobic activity or a hot bath to warm your muscles before stretching. Neuromotor exercises: • Neuromotor exercises (sometimes called "functional fitness training") are recommended for 2 or 3 days per week. • Exercises should involve motor skills (balance, agility, coordination, and gait), *proprioceptive exercise* training and multifaceted activities (e.g., tai chi and yoga) to improve physical function and to prevent falls in older adults. • 20 to 30 minutes each day is appropriate for neuromotor exercise.

As you can see from Table 9-2, there are many sets of recommendations; it can be difficult to understand which is best for you. The goal is to be active. A great way to get started is to determine what you currently do. Think back to the SMART goals we discussed earlier in this chapter (Specific, Measurable, Attainable, Realistic, and Time-sensitive). If you have not exercised in years and struggle with joint pain it is unwise and unrealistic for you to begin with a 30-minute jog. Start slowly and gradually increase the amount of movement your body is able to tolerate. The first week you might aim to be active 2 to 3 days with 15 minutes of walking, and then gradually increase your effort to 20 minutes, and then 25 minutes, 4 days a week, and then 30 minutes in each episode. Exercising with a partner is a great way to stay motivated. Try asking a friend to go on a pre-dinner walk with you a few nights a week. If you have access to a gym, plan to meet your friend and try out the stationary bikes to get the day started. As you establish your fitness goals you will learn how often you should exercise. You will want to create a plan that works for you over the long term.

What Kind of Exercise Should I Do?

Health-related physical fitness for people with obesity includes three components: cardio-respiratory fitness, adjustment of body composition, and muscular fitness (https://www.ncbi.nlm.nih.gov/pmc/articles/PMC3096271/). Cardiovascular activity helps achieve heart health and decrease cholesterol levels and high blood pressure. Muscular fitness increases muscle strength while decreasing fat to improve body composition. You want to include cardiovascular and muscle-building exercise into your exercise routine. Cardiorespiratory fitness or cardiovascular endurance refers to how well your body is able to deliver oxygen to your body tissues. Basically, you want to be able to move oxygen to your muscles and not become short of breath. There are many types of cardiovascular activities (e.g., walking, water activities, biking, seated aerobics). Be mindful of any joint pain, and aim for non-weight bearing activities (e.g., recumbent cycling, using portable pedalers, seated aerobics, or water activities) if you are having problems. Remember to start slowly, possibly with 10 minutes of exercise and then slowly increase the duration of your exercise. Exercise at a pace that allows you to hold a conversation without too much difficulty. Get involved in an activity that you enjoy. If you enjoy dancing, try a Zumba® or dance class. If you enjoy sports, consider joining a basketball team or find a basketball court for shooting and playing.

Improving body compositions refers to increasing lean muscle mass and decreasing body fat percentages. As you increase your muscle mass, your body will burn more energy and it will improve your health. Muscular fitness allows a muscle or muscle group to perform continuously without fatigue. Activities for muscle fitness include calisthenics, weight training, and certain cardio activities.

Should I Attempt to Stop Drinking Alcohol or Smoking Cigarettes?

Alcohol is not calorie-free and use of it might interfere with some of your medications. Consult your physician if alcohol is contraindicated with use of any of your medications or with your health conditions; stop drinking alcohol if it is. Take a moment and reflect on how much alcohol you are drinking. Drinking in moderation is considered one drink per day for women and two drinks daily for men. A drink is considered as 12 ounces of beer, 5 ounces of wine, or 1.5 ounces of hard liquor. On average, regular beer provides 146 calories per bottle, whereas light beer provides 99 calories. Liquor provides an average of 97 calories per drink, not including a mixer, such as soda or juice, which would increase the total calories in the drink. Wine provides 105 to 125 calories per serving, depending on the type consumed. If you are drinking more than moderate amounts, you might want to consider decreasing your intake. Many people find that when they are intoxicated they consume more snacks and increase their overall calorie intake. Keep in mind that alcoholic beverages add to your daily calorie intake and might be a ready target for decreasing your intake of calories.

One study found that with obesity, smokers have a life expectancy 13 years less than normal-weight non-smokers (http://ajcn.nutrition.org/content/87/4/801.full). Smoking increases the risk of cardiovascular disease and metabolic syndrome (which involves weight gain, abnormal glucose levels, and elevated cholesterol levels). Many people are fearful that if they quit smoking they will gain weight. Studies show that the benefits of smoking cessation outweigh the risk of additional weight gain. Deciding to quit smoking is a huge step in taking care of your body. There are many programs that offer support when attempting to stop smoking. The Centers for Disease Control and Prevention (CDC) has a program to assist you in creating a Quit Plan; providing suggestions on how to help you manage your cravings; various support options, such as SmokefreeTxt; or an opportunity to chat with a counselor. Be mindful to incorporate balanced eating and physical activity to combat weight gain. Drink adequate fluids and eat on a schedule. People who have smoked for years might find that they miss the hand-to-mouth habit. Be proactive and identify strategies to prevent your replacing food with cigarettes. Experiment with brushing your teeth after meals or chewing sugar-free gum or mints. Keep your hands busy by taking up knitting or crocheting, beadwork, origami, or keep a pen or pencil in your hand, or try a fidget toy or a stress ball. A support system can be helpful. Reach out for help when you are craving a cigarette.

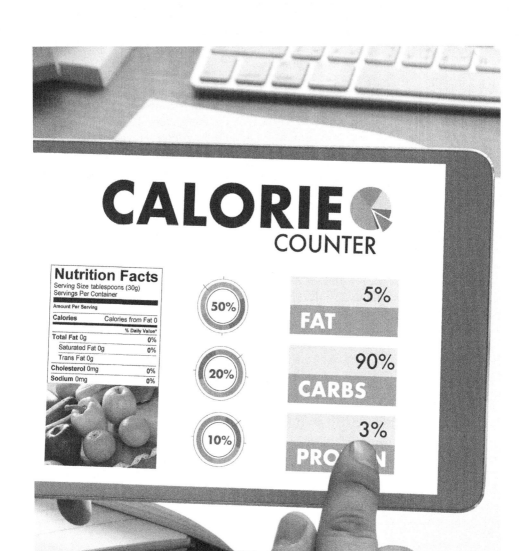

WEIGHT-LOSS PROGRAMS
Kim George, MS, RD, LD

CHAPTER

In This Chapter

- Acid Alkaline Diet

- The Atkins Diet

- Weight Watchers

- The Jenny Craig Diet

- The Cabbage Soup Diet

- The Paleo Diet

- Whole30 Program

- The Nutrisystem Diet

- The Slim-Fast Diet

- The Glycemic Index Diet

- The Macrobiotic Diet

- The Ornish Diet

- The Pritikin Principle

- The South Beach Diet

- The Zone Diet

Introduction

Commercial weight-loss programs and fad diets are abundant; they appear to be every-where you look (Figure 10-1). Not uncommonly, people become desperate to lose weight and they explore commercial and fad diets to aid in losing weight. Unfortunately, finding reliable information about diets and their purported health benefits is a challenge. Few of these weight-loss programs are ever examined using the scientific rigor normally expended on health interventions involving the public (i.e., *double-blind placebo-controlled studies* for medicines or surgical interventions seeking *US Food and Drug Administration* [FDA] approval). Diet websites are often difficult to navigate and often demand that you sign up (and pay) for their programs before you can learn more about them. Ultimately, the goal of this chapter is more about understanding the importance of eating a balanced meal across food groups, learning about portion control, and becoming flexible than it is to impart knowledge about specific diets. Diets that promise quick weight loss might be eye-catching, but they often overlook the principles of long-term, sustainable, healthy eating.

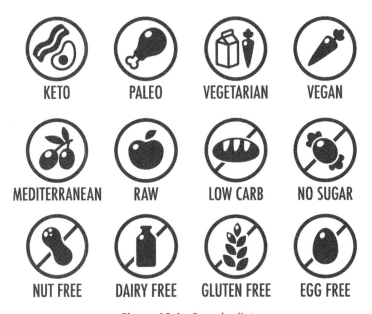

KETO   PALEO   VEGETARIAN   VEGAN

MEDITERRANEAN   RAW   LOW CARB   NO SUGAR

NUT FREE   DAIRY FREE   GLUTEN FREE   EGG FREE

Figure 10-1: Sample diets.

Acid Alkaline Diet

Background

The *Acid Alkaline Diet* focuses on controlling your *pH* through your diet to achieve health, weight loss, disease prevention, and overall health. The diet explains that foods (such as meat, wheat, refined sugar, and processed foods) produce acids that lead to poor health. Therefore, the dieter should eat alkaline foods to protect against disease and weight gain. One measure of acidity and alkalinity throughout the body is the pH (calculated on a 0 to 14 scale). Acidic substances are scored from 0 to 7. Alkaline substances are scored from 7 to 14. The diet encourages at least a 60/40 alkaline to acidic mix to maintain and promote a healthy balance. The dieter will need to understand where foods fall on the acid/alkaline scale and refer to the "Acid Alkaline Diet for Dummies" for guidance. The diet encourages you to build meals and snacks around fruits and vegetables instead of meats and starches for an alkaline balance. Examples of alkaline foods include fruits and vegetables (http://www.webmd.com/food-recipes/ss/slideshow-exotic-fruits), soybeans and tofu, as well as some nuts, seeds, and legumes. The dieter should aim for foods higher in alkaline content. Acid-forming foods include dairy, eggs, meat, yeast, wheat products, alcohol, caffeine, and processed foods.

Professional Review

The Acid Alkaline Diet is a non-scientific approach. The foods we eat will not affect our blood pH. Many dieters will benefit from increasing their fruit and vegetable intake but they also need to consume adequate amounts of protein and whole grains. This diet is restrictive and puts the dieter at risk for nutritional deficiencies.

The Atkins Diet

Background

The *Atkins Diet* is a classic low-carbohydrate diet promoted by Dr. Robert Atkins. The diet states that it can "flip the body's metabolic switch" from burning carbohydrates to burning fat. There are four phases with increased carbohydrates as the phases progress. The Atkins diet has an extensive website that you can visit at (https://www.atkins.com/how-it-works).

The first phase (or Introduction Phase) states that it will "jump start your metabolism." Phase 1 lasts for at least 2 weeks and the dieter decreases "net carbs" to 20 grams daily.

During Phase 2 (or the Balancing Phase) the dieter "finds their personal carb balance." New foods (such as nuts, seeds, strawberries, blueberries, melon, cottage cheese, and yogurt) are added. "Net carbs" are started at 25 grams and increased to between 30 and 80 grams.

Phase 3 begins as the dieter is 10 pounds away from their goal weight. This stage is designed for fine-tuning the diet and allows the dieter to focus on maintaining their weight loss. In Phase 3, the daily Net Carb intake increases gradually. After weight loss is maintained for a month, the dieter moves into Phase 4.

Phase 4 (or Lifetime Maintenance) advertises itself as a permanent lifestyle.

Professional Review

Many dieters who follow the Atkins diet find that they are able to lose weight quickly. As with many fad diets, people have a difficult time continuing with this plan over the long term. Dieters might lack an understanding on how to move throughout the phases. However, the plan does not allow the dieter to enjoy a variety of foods and the recommended portion sizes in the foods throughout the four phases are small. It is difficult to achieve adequate nutrition while following this diet. The Institute of Medicine report "Dietary Reference Intakes for Energy, Carbohydrate, Fiber, Fat, Fatty Acids, Cholesterol, Protein, and Amino Acids" (IOM, 2002) established a Recommended Dietary Allowance (RDA) for carbohydrate of 130 grams per day for adults and children. Both Phase 1 and 2 of the Atkins Diet encouraged as little as 20 grams of carbohydrates per day and as much as 80 grams of carbohydrates (or 15%–62%) of the recommended intake of carbohydrates. Carbohydrates are essential for your *central nervous system* (CNS) and they provide your body with quick energy. Inadequate intake of carbohydrates will affect your brain health. It is recommended that at least half of your calories come from carbohydrates. As you restrict carbohydrates you are also restricting fiber intake, which is necessary for blood sugar control and satiety; carbohydrates also assist with decreasing *cholesterol* and aid in regular bowel functions. Nutritionally, your body would be at risk if you decided to follow the Atkins diet.

Weight Watchers

Background

Weight Watchers focuses on balance; it uses a group setting for a support system. The newest program, *Beyond the Scale*, encourages the dieter to make better food choices, to move their body more, and to shift their diet mindset. The program is designed to assist in weight loss but also to focus on benefits other than weight by balancing nutrition and fitness. Members are assigned a certain number of points daily (based on their age, gender, height, weight, and whether they desire weight loss or to maintain their weight). There are extra weekly points that range from 14 to 42 depending on the individual and their specific plan. The method of calculating points has changed throughout the years; currently, it uses SmartPoints. Each food and beverage is allocated SmartPoints based on calories and on the content of saturated fat, sugar, and protein. The point system does not encourage you to avoid any food, but it calculates points based on portion sizes. A higher calorie and fat food item would accrue more points and leave the dieter with fewer points to use during the rest of the day.

Weight Watchers has different types of programs. You have the option of going to meetings, participating only on-line, or to have a personal coach. Memberships costs vary based on their location. A 3-month subscription for On-line Plus can cost $3.07/week, meetings can cost $6.92/week, and Coaching can cost $8.46/week. Lifetime membership is earned by members who reach and maintain a weight goal that falls within the parameters of the Healthy Weight Ranges; it is free for meetings members.

Professional Review

The Weight Watchers program encourages balance and teaches members that all foods can fit into your diet. The program comes at a cost, and members might find it too costly to continue over the long term. The program allows the member to eat as many fruits and non-starchy vegetables as desired, and the member must keep in mind that these foods are a great source of fiber and nutrients, but they are not calorie free. The calorie content of the fruits and vegetables can add up throughout the day. Calculating points for each food item you eat can be difficult and time consuming. The program can serve as an educational tool for a person who wants to understand how to balance their nutrition and their exercise.

For example, I had a client, Lucy, who tried Weight Watchers to help her lose weight after she delivered her son. She used the program religiously and began to understand portion size. She learned how to enjoy a cupcake and to balance her points for the rest of the day. The problem arose when she did not have a label for a food item and could not calculate how many points she was eating. She had a weekly meeting at work at which she and her co-workers frequently brought in snacks. Prior to the meetings she felt anxious about not knowing what would be in the meeting and how many points to allot for what was available. She would find herself distracted in the meeting and would either avoid the snacks altogether or eat past her fullness. Her frustration with her inability to eat unplanned or unknown foods eventually led her to stop the program.

The Jenny Craig Diet

Background

The *Jenny Craig Diet* is a calorie-controlled diet program with pre-packed meals. The dieter has the choice of two programs: in-center (in which you have personal meetings and regular visits with a consultant) or at-home (with on-line resources with phone or video chat). There are three levels within the program. The first level involves adjusting to the program by eating the foods in small portions. The second level adds physical activity, and during the third level, dieters work on weight-loss maintenance. The dieters' plans vary from 1,200 to 2,300 calories per day based on the participants current weight, fitness habits, and motivation. A personal consultant guides the dieter weekly with regard to nutrition and exercise. The meals are pre-packaged for portion control, and the dieter provides their own fruits, vegetables, and dairy items. After the dieter is halfway to their goal weight, they will transition back to preparing their own meals using Jenny's recipes. The price of the program and meals vary, but it can cost $525 to $705 per month; $14.99 per month with $25 enrollment fee with no access to a health consultant, $19.99 plus an $99 for an enrollment fee with up to three consultations a week, or $39.99 with no enrollment fee for a weekly consultation. The average cost daily is $15 to $23.

Professional Review

The program is easy to follow with the pre-portioned meals, but it can be difficult for the dieter when they adjust to eating out or to cooking on their own. The cost of the plan can be significant for the dieter. Dieters might find it difficult to eat with family or loved ones due to having individual meals while following the pre-packaged meals.

The Cabbage Soup Diet

Background

The *Cabbage Soup Diet* claims to help you lose 10 pounds or more in a week. There are several recipes available on-line for the Cabbage Soup Diet. The website states that it is not suitable for long-term weight loss but is designed for kick-starting dieting. It is not recommended for more than 7 days and you should not start the diet again for at least 2 weeks after completion. It cautions against high-intensity workouts. You are permitted to eat fat-free cabbage soup two to three times a day with other permitted foods as follows:

- Day 1—Consume all of the fruits (except bananas) you desire. You can also eat the soup. You can drink unsweetened teas, cranberry juice, and water.

- Day 2—Consume non-starchy vegetables during the day, and you can "reward" yourself with a plain baked potato for dinner. Although you can't eat fruit on this day, you can have the soup as desired.

- Day 3—You may mix the foods used on days one and two with fruits and vegetables, but not eat a baked potato. You can eat the soup as desired.

- Day 4—Consume bananas (up to eight) and as many glasses of skim milk as desired. This day is designed to help decrease your desire for sweets. You can eat the soup as desired.

- Day 5—Consume up to 20 ounces of beef or skinless baked chicken and up to eight tomatoes. Eat your soup at least once on this day.

- Day 6—You can eat all the beef and vegetables desired. You should not have a baked potato today, but you can have at least one portion of soup.

- Day 7—Consume all the brown rice, unsweetened fruit juices, vegetables, and soup you desire.

- Day 8—Begin a moderate long-term eating plan.

Professional Review

The Cabbage Soup diet does not provide adequate nutrients for the dieter. The dieter might have low energy levels and find it difficult to concentrate and to think. It can be dangerous if a dieter participates in exercise due to the inadequate nutrient intake, and the participant is at risk of fainting or experiencing other medical issues. The diet does not teach the participant about balanced eating, and quick weight loss might be related to fluid loss more than fat loss. The inadequate protein might aid in more muscle loss than desired. We do not recommend that you follow this fad diet. The recommended schedule of the diet does not align with any nutritional guidelines.

On a personal note, while I was growing up, my best friend's father followed the Cabbage Soup Diet a few times each year. I remember walking into my friend's kitchen and smelling the strong, pungent smell of cabbage soup. Their refrigerator would be filled with soup containers. I can still picture him, a large man who had played college football, eating a bowl of cabbage soup for dinner. After a few days of following the diet he would become short-tempered. Looking back, I imagine that his blood sugar must have been low and his tolerance for teenage girls was at a minimum. At the end of the diet, which invariably did not last the full seven days, we would join him in a meal with large fried pork chops, mashed potatoes with gravy, rolls, and corn. Then, we would have the chore of throwing out the containers of uneaten cabbage soup!

The Paleo Diet

Background

The *Paleo Diet* states that it is based upon every day, modern foods that mimic the food groups of our pre-agricultural, hunter-gatherer, ancestors. The diet explains that there are seven fundamental characteristics of hunter-gatherer diets that will help to optimize your health, minimize your risk of chronic disease, and lose weight:

- Higher protein intake

- Lower carbohydrate intake and lower glycemic index

- Higher fiber intake

- Moderate to higher fat intake dominated by monounsaturated and polyunsaturated fats with balanced omega-3 and omega-6 fats

- Higher potassium and lower sodium intake

- Net dietary alkaline load that balances dietary acid

- Higher intake of vitamins, minerals, *anti-oxidants*, and plant phytochemicals

The diet does not allow cereal grains, legumes, dairy, refined sugar, potatoes, processed foods, refined vegetable oil, or salt.

The diet does allow grass-produced meat, fish and seafood, fresh fruits and vegetables, eggs, nuts and seeds, and healthful oil.

Professional Review

The Paleo Diet advertises loose scientific claims. People would benefit from increased fiber but the diet encourages the dieter to avoid whole grains. Whole grains are proven to provide the body with key nutrients, such as fiber and carbohydrates, which are needed for brain health. The diet is restrictive and encourages the dieter to avoid dairy which provides a person with calcium, vitamin D, protein, and B-vitamins. Dairy is prohibited but the diet offers potassium, calcium, vitamin D, B-vitamins, and protein. Our pre-agricultural, hunter-gatherer ancestors ate what was available to them, and their intake was dependent on what they could hunt and gather at any particular moment. They might have eaten more protein when they were able to hunt wildlife, and more fruits when they were in areas with fruit trees.

Whole30 Program

Background

The *Whole30 Program* states that certain foods (such as sugar, grains, dairy, and legumes) have a negative impact on your health. It encourages a dieter to avoid these food items to allow the body to heal and to recover from damage. The program states that it is not a diet but that it is designed to "change your life," by eliminating cravings, rebalancing hormones, curing digestive issues, improving medical conditions, and boosting energy and immune function. The diet allows moderate portions of meat, seafood, and eggs; lots of vegetables;

some fruit; plenty of natural fats; and herbs, spices, and seasonings. The diet does not permit added sugar or artificial sugar, alcohol, grains, legumes, dairy, carrageenan, monosodium glutamate (MSG), sulfites, baked goods, or junk foods. Participants are encouraged not to weigh themselves for 30 days.

Professional Review

The Whole30 Program is a restrictive method of eating. The plan states that food is the cause of many medical conditions, but a variety of foods is essential to provide our bodies with adequate and varied nutrients. Unless there is a medical reason or allergy, it is not prudent to avoid an entire food group, much less multiple food groups.

I had a client, George, an athlete who learned about Whole30 from his workout buddies and he decided to try it. He wanted to maximize his health and felt that this method of eating would be a great addition. During the first few days of the diet he felt great and was proud of himself for avoiding processed foods and increasing his vegetable intake. As time progressed, he noticed increased hunger at night and started snacking on cubes of chicken. He enjoyed eating out with friends a few times a week but he began to meet with friends after meals because cooking at home was easier and he knew all the ingredients he was eating. He had lunch meetings at work at which he would ask the waiter for double protein portions and to replace the starch with a non-starchy vegetable. These requests often made his colleagues take a second look at him. After a couple of months, he recognized that he had rearranged his work and social calendar to better accommodate his new manner of eating. He decided his relationships were more important than a method of eating and he reincorporated dairy, and grains, and he no longer had to read labels on all of the foods he ate. He could be more flexible with his evening snack and switch from cubes of chicken to cheese and crackers. He learned from the Whole30 program that he was not eating enough vegetables before and he continued this new habit, but he no longer had to meet friends after dinner to watch sporting events.

The Nutrisystem Diet

Background

The *Nutrisystem Diet* is a home-delivered pre-packaged meal program. The *Lean 13 Plan* claims that women will lose up to 13 pounds and 7 inches off their waist in the first month, whereas men can expect to lose 15 pounds and 7 inches off their waist. There is a "Turbo Take Off Week" during which the dieter eats 1,000 calories to enhance weight loss. The program prepares and delivers meals and outlines what to eat and when to eat it. The dieter is encouraged to avoid high glycemic index foods and alcohol. The plan has the dieter eat three meals with two snacks and a dessert snack from pre-packaged options. The dieter adds their personal selections of fruits and vegetables, protein, and dairy. There are three choices with a 4-week plan.

- Basic—Start the first month with the Turbo10 plan and then receive portion-controlled meals as well as access to on-line tools and trackers.

- Core—Start the first month with the Turbo10 plan and then receive portion-controlled meals, access to on-line tools, trackers, and diet counselors on call.

- Uniquely Yours—Start the first month with the Turbo10 plan and then receive portion-controlled meals, including Nutrisystem's new premium frozen cuisine. The dieter has access to on-line tools, trackers, and diet counselors on call.

Basic starts at $9.82/day or $274.99 for 4 weeks with free shipping, whereas the Core plan is the most popular at $10.54/day or $294.99 for 4 weeks with free shipping, and the Uniquely Yours plan starts at $11.96/day or $334.99 for 4 weeks.

Professional Review

The diet is pre-packaged and helps the dieter with portion-control for weight loss. The Turbo 10 plan provides inadequate calories to support a healthy brain and body functions. The dieter has a limited ability to eat with friends and family due to the pre-packaged meals. The cost can be a hindrance, and the dieter might become tired of eating packaged foods. The diet does not provide the dieter with education, and when the dieter stops eating the pre-packed meals, they have not gained knowledge on how to continue or to maintain their weight loss with every-day foods.

I have worked with clients who tried Nutrisystem, and they felt that they were able to lose weight only if they followed the program with pre-portioned meals. Each time they stopped the program they gained back the weight and felt hopeless with weight loss. The program would be more beneficial to a dieter if it provided the dieter with education to support balanced eating and weight loss. Education is the equivalent of gold for lifestyle changes.

The Slim-Fast Diet

Background

The *Slim-Fast Diet* is a 1,200-calorie plan. The dieter prepares one 500 calorie meal a day, consumes two slim-fast meal replacements via a bar or shake, and three snacks. The diet claims to facilitate 1 to 2 pounds of weight loss per week. The Slim-Fast products' prices vary but are available via a 30-day supply of six boxes of meal bars, five boxes of snack bars, and 32 shake mixes; it costs $75, plus shipping. A five-pack of meal bars runs about $4.88; a six-pack of snack bars is $3.25; an eight-pack of pre-made shakes is $9.88; and a carton of protein powder shake mix is $8.

Professional Review

Dieters have unique calorie needs for weight loss. A man weighing 350 pounds requires more calories to support basic bodily functions than does a woman weighing 250 pounds. An equal amount of food is not necessarily appropriate for two different people. Weight loss is achieved due to the low calorie content of shakes and snacks. The dieter can become tired of eating pre-packaged snacks, shakes, and bars.

The Glycemic Index Diet

Background

The glycemic index categorizes carbohydrates as "good" or "bad." Carbohydrates are a ranked on a scale from 0 to 100 based on how much they increase blood sugar levels after eating. Bad carbohydrates are said to increase blood sugar more quickly, to leave the person hungrier sooner, and to have a higher glycemic index. Good carbohydrates are lower on the glycemic index scale and are said to aid the dieter into feeling fuller longer. The dieter is encouraged to eat low-glycemic index carbohydrates (with a glycemic index of 55 or lower), to eat less medium-glycemic index carbohydrates (56 to 69), and to limit high-glycemic index carbohydrates (70 and higher).

Professional Review

The glycemic index encourages ingestion of higher-fiber foods that provide the body with many benefits, such as blood sugar stability, satiety, heart health, and regular bowel movements. However, the portions of foods tested for their glycemic index are not typical portion sizes. Most people eat several different types of food (such as a turkey and cheese sandwich with a side of carrot sticks) at once, which changes the glycemic index of the food items entirely. The glycemic index varies based on where the food is grown and how ripe the food is when it is consumed. The glycemic index is also difficult to understand. The dieter must look up each food individually. The glycemic index is completely independent of the nutrition value of the food item and it focuses on how quickly blood sugar rises when the food is eaten alone.

I had a client, Maria, who had diabetes; her doctor encouraged her to follow the glycemic index. During an appointment, we discussed various non-starchy vegetable options that she could add to her meals. I suggested carrots and she adamantly told me, "No, carrots were not good for a person with diabetes." A cup of carrots provides around 6 grams of carbohydrate and a cup of broccoli has around 5 grams of carbohydrate. For comparison, a half cup of rice or potatoes has around 20 grams of carbohydrates. The glycemic index of carrots is 92 categorizing it as a high-glycemic-index food. The glycemic index of broccoli is 0 categorizing it has as a low glycemic index food. Carbohydrates are a main driver of blood sugar, and 5 to 6 grams of carbohydrates are considered a non-starchy vegetable and do not increase blood sugar rapidly or even much at all. It saddens me to think people who follow the glycemic index are missing out on foods they enjoy based on loose science.

The Macrobiotic Diet

Background

The *Macrobiotic Diet* is an approach to help the dieter identify what foods are right for them to achieve balance and overall health and happiness. The diet follows the Chinese principle of balance, known as *yin* and *yang*. The macrobiotic diet claims to assist in warding off and curing diseases. The diet encourages organic, locally grown foods, and limits processed and chemical-containing foods. Dieters are encouraged to eat regularly, chew their food well, listen to their bodies, and stay active. The diet recommends that 40% to 60% of a daily diet include organic whole grains, 20% to 30% locally grown vegetables, and 5% to 10% beans and bean products (such as tofu, miso, and tempeh), and sea vegetables (like seaweed, nori, and agar). The dieter can consume fresh fish and seafood, locally grown fruit, pickles, and nuts, several times a week. The dieter is discouraged from eating dairy, eggs, poultry, processed foods, refined sugars and meats, tropical fruits, fruit juice, and certain vegetables (such as asparagus, eggplant, spinach, tomatoes, and zucchini). The dieter must drink only when thirsty and should avoid spicy foods, strong alcoholic beverages (http://www.webmd.com/mental-health/addiction/understanding-alcohol-abuse-basics), soda, coffee, and foods that are refined, processed, or chemically preserved. The macrobiotic approach encourages the dieter to chew at least 50 times, pause and give gratitude for your food before eating, eat two to three times a day, and stop eating before you are full. The Kushi Institute is a resource for coaching from macrobiotic counselors.

Professional Review

The diet encourages use of whole foods with a focus on whole grains, fruits, and vegetables. These are foods that many people could eat more. The diet is restrictive and avoids food groups that provide the body with key nutrients. This dieter is at risk for B_{12} and vitamin D deficiencies. The diet is difficult to follow and requires research and commitment.

The Ornish Diet

Background

With the *Ornish Diet*, as noted in his book, *The Spectrum*, Dr. Dean Ornish encourages nutrition, exercise, stress management, and emotional support options to aid in weight loss or curing chronic diseases. Foods are categorized into five groups (from group one which is the healthiest to group five with the least healthy foods). It recommends that more foods from group one be eaten for increased health benefits. The diet encourages decreasing high-fat animal proteins while increasing fruits, vegetables, whole grains, legumes, non-fat dairy, soy products, and egg whites. Moderate amounts of fish, skinless chicken, avocados, nuts, and seeds should be eaten. No more than 10% of calories should be consumed from fat and only eaten in foods that naturally contain fats. Nuts should be limited to very small portions because of their high fat content. Cholesterol should be limited to 10 milligrams or less per day. This is achieved when dairy is limited to two non-fat dairy products daily; dairy alternatives such as soy milk are encouraged. The diet encourages plant-based proteins (such as egg whites, tofu, tempeh, beans, legumes, non-fat cheese, and non-fat yogurt). Foods should be flavored with spices, herbs, and other natural flavor enhancers (such as citrus and vinegars). Stimulants, such as caffeine, should be limited to promote balance, calmness, and a peaceful way of living. Green tea may be consumed (up to two cups daily), whereas caffeinated coffee is limited to one cup or less, and up to two cups of decaffeinated or up to two cups of black tea per day are permitted. Dr. Ornish states that food is not all-or-nothing; he focuses on eating the right foods. The dieter is encouraged to focus on foods found in nature while limiting processed foods. Calories are limited only if the dieter is trying to lose weight. If weight loss is desired, the dieter should eat small, frequent meals throughout the day with portion control. "Bad carbs" (such as refined carbohydrates, sugar, concentrated sweeteners, white flour, and white rice) should be limited in the dieter's intake.

Sugar is not recommended, but it can be eaten in moderation, whereas added sugar (via maple syrup, agave, honey, white or brown sugar along with non-fat sweets, and refined carbohydrates) are limited to no more than two servings per day. Alcohol is not encouraged, but one serving daily is allowed.

Dr. Ornish recommends aerobic activities, resistance training, and flexibility. He also encourages deep breathing, yoga, and meditation to manage stress, and encourages dieters to spend time with loved ones. He explains how to lose weight, improve cholesterol and blood pressure, prevent and reverse type 2 diabetes, heart disease, prostate cancer, and breast cancer.

Professional Review

The diet encourages use of fiber-rich foods, and many people can benefit from increasing their fiber. The Ornish Diet is difficult to follow due to the recommendation of 10% of calories from fat. The USDA recommends 20% to 35% of calories from fat. Fat is necessary to aid in absorption of fat soluble vitamins A, D, E and K, it assists in satiety, insulates organs, promotes brain health, and adds flavor to foods. As a person decreases fat intake, they typically increase their carbohydrate intake.

The Pritikin Principle

Background

The *Pritikin Program* is a low-fat, high-fiber plan that encourages exercise to prevent or cure heart disease. Fat intake is limited to 10% of daily calories. The diet encourages fruits, vegetables, low-fat dairy, legumes, lean protein, and fish. The dieter aims to limit oils, refined sugars, salt, and refined grains. The plan recommends avoiding processed meats, foods high in saturated fat (http://www.webmd.com/cholesterol-management/features/truth-about-saturated-fats), and those made with trans fat (http://www.webmd.com/food-recipes/understanding-trans-fats), organ meats, processed meats, and high-cholesterol foods (http://www.webmd.com/cholesterol-management/default.htm) like eggs.

There are 10 steps to *The Pritikin Edge*.

1. Start each meal with soup, salad, fruit, or whole grains. It is said to promote fullness.

2. Avoid high-calorie drinks, especially soda. A glass of wine each day can be good for the heart, but you should skip most alcoholic beverages.

3. Avoid high-calorie foods.

4. Snack at set times and only on healthy foods.

5. Choose whole, unprocessed foods as often as possible, and always avoid fast food.

6. Exercise regularly, combining lots of walking with strength training.

7. Go easy on eating meat, especially red meat. Instead, opt for fatty fish, like salmon.

8. Skip extra salt.

9. Don't smoke.

10. Ease stress.

For support the dieter can sign up for a free newsletter and seek on-line support. A starter kit is available at $459.95 and includes the "One-Week Pritikin Frozen Food Plan," a One-Year On-line Pritikin Membership, and the book *The Pritikin Edge: 10 Essential Ingredients for a Long and Delicious Life*. After the introduction, meal plans are $225 a week. Dieters are strongly encouraged to visit the Florida-based Pritikin Longevity Center and Spa, where prices range from $4,000 a week in the summer to $6,000 a week during the winter.

Professional Review

The diet is restrictive and difficult to comply with over the long term. As with the Ornish diet the recommended fat intake is very low. Fat is necessary for health. The diet has some balanced recommendations including aiming for whole foods and limiting processed foods, but it leaves the dieter with limited flexibility.

The South Beach Diet

Background

The *South Beach Diet* is a low-carbohydrate, high-protein, and healthy-fat diet. The diet claims that the dieter can lose 8 to 13 pounds during the first two weeks, and then 1 to 2 pounds each week thereafter. The diet uses the glycemic index to determine good and bad carbohydrates. The diet states that foods with a high glycemic index increase your blood sugar faster than foods with a lower glycemic index. The diet explains that the increase in blood sugar can increase your appetite and cause weight gain and can even lead to diabetes or heart disease. The diet encourages use of mono-unsaturated fats and focuses on the benefits of fiber consumed via whole grains, fruits, and vegetables. The dieter does not need to count calories, fat grams, or carbohydrates. The plan encourages eating three meals a day with two snacks. The diet consists of three phases.

Phase 1 is designed to "jump start" weight loss and decrease cravings for sugar and refined starches. This phase lasts two weeks. The dieter is encouraged to avoid all foods with a high glycemic index. The dieter is permitted to eat non-starchy vegetables, lean protein, and foods with unsaturated fats. The dieter cannot eat starches, fruit, juice, or consume alcohol. The dieter eats 4.5 cups of vegetables and 2 cups of milk or dairy each day. The dieter may start with 2 ounces of protein at breakfast and 3 ounces for lunch and dinner and is encouraged to eat slowly and return for seconds if hunger persists.

Phase 2 is the long-term weight-loss phase. The dieter can slowly reintroduce "healthy" carbohydrates (such as whole grains, fruit, and more starchy vegetables). The dieter consumes three servings of fruit and three servings of starches per day. Two daily snacks are optional and a glass of wine at dinner is permitted. Weight loss is advertised at 1 to 2 pounds a week, and this phase will continue until the dieter reaches their goal weight.

Phase 3 is a maintenance phase. All foods are permitted, but if the dieter develops cravings or gains weight they are advised to return to Phase 1 or 2. The South Beach Diet On-line offers tools to track weight, recipes, an option for a customized meal plan, dining-out guides, and community support. Membership is $4 per week, but the first 7 days are free. An optional on-line membership is $5 per week. The diet has evolved over time and now recommends exercise as an important part of your lifestyle. The South Beach Diet says that regular exercise will boost your metabolism and help prevent weight-loss plateaus.

Professional Review

Phase 1 encourages an inadequate carbohydrate intake. Carbohydrates are necessary for health and they provide your brain with energy for optimal thinking. The diet contains many rules and does not teach the dieter about balance; instead, it applies all or nothing principles.

The Zone Diet

Background

The *Zone Diet* states that the key to weight loss is achieving proper hormonal balance and keeping your blood sugar stable. The creator, Barry Sears, believes that to ensure that your insulin and other inflammation-promoting hormone levels stay "in the zone," you should eat foods in the correct proportions at every meal: 40% carbohydrates, 30% protein, and 30% fat. The diet advertises that when the dieter follows the guidelines, they will lose 1 to 2 pounds weekly. The Zone Diet typically provides 1,200 calories daily for women and 1,500 calories daily for men. The dieter will eat five times a day with three meals and two snacks. Breakfast needs to be eaten within one hour of waking up followed by snacks and meals every five hours. The dinner plate should be divided into three equal sections of a lean protein (about the size of the person's hand) and the other two sections should have colorful carbohydrates (such a fruit and a vegetable). A healthy fat (such as olive oil, almonds, or an avocado) will round out the meal. The diet does not prohibit foods but encourages certain types. Lean proteins (such as skinless chicken, turkey, fish, egg whites, low-fat dairy, tofu, and soy meat substitutes) are encouraged. Carbohydrates are categorized as "good" or "bad," and the dieter should aim for low-glycemic carbohydrates. Low-glycemic carbohydrates are said to keep blood sugar and metabolism stable and to promote satiety while higher-glycemic carbohydrates increase hunger and promote unstable blood sugar levels. The diet encourages vegetables other than corn and carrots, and fruits other than bananas and raisins. The dieter should avoid pasta, bread, bagels, cereals, and potatoes. Small amounts of healthy fats are added to each meal; the dieter should avoid fatty red meat, egg yolks, liver and other organ meats, and processed foods. The dieter can seek resources via on-line membership at zonediet.com. Sears states that exercise is more important for weight maintenance than it is for weight loss.

Professional Review

The Zone Diet is a restrictive and complicated diet. The recommended calorie levels are inadequate for many men and women. Dieters must ensure that they consume adequate energy to fuel their bodies. Even though a dieter will want to decrease their calorie intake, they do not want to starve their bodies. This diet does not provide a dieter with valuable nutrition education and is not likely to build a long-term method of eating.

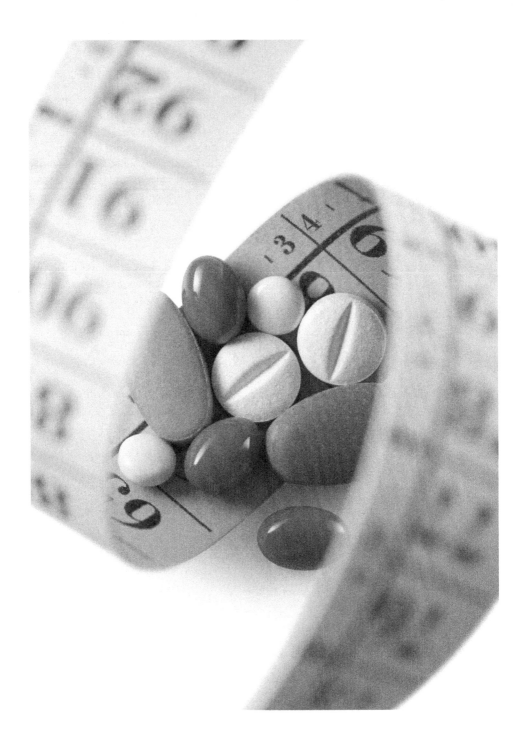

WHAT MEDICATIONS CAN HELP ME LOSE WEIGHT?

Sherry Grogan, APRN, PMHNP-BC and
Jonathan R. Stevens, MD, MPH

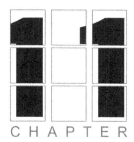

C H A P T E R

In This Chapter

- Which Medications Can Facilitate Weight Loss?

- How Do These Medications Work?

- What Side Effects Do Anti-Obesity Medications Have?

- What Over-The-Counter Weight-Loss Medications Are Available and Should I Use Them?

Which Medications Can Facilitate Weight Loss?

"I've tried everything, and I just can't keep the weight off." How often have you felt this way? You've tried multiple diets, reduced your calories, eaten your veggies, worked out faithfully at the gym, taken the stairs instead of the elevator—and yet nothing seems to change, especially over the long term. As we've discussed in earlier chapters, there are multiple reasons why it can be difficult to lose weight, including our body's own desire to maintain the status quo. Several theories try to account for why it's so difficult to lose and to maintain weight. Our brain controls both our energy intake and expenditure through complex signaling of our nervous system with *neurotransmitters, endorphins, hormones*, reward systems of pleasurable stimuli in the *mesocorticolimbic dopamine systems*, and through feedback loops with signals, such as *leptin* and *ghrelin*. People with obesity have a variety of ways in which they respond to hunger and to satiety cues as well as emotional and reward cues, compared to those who are not obese (Yanowski & Yanowski, 2014). Certainly, there are strong behavioral components, such as eating more calories than needed, losing motivation to maintain a restrictive diet, and failing to exercise regularly. Other factors, including biological factors such as your metabolism slowing down (adaptive thermogenesis) and your hunger increasing, are also involved. There are reductions in leptin and *cholecystokinin*, and increases in ghrelin. This is our body's way of maintaining a balance (*homeostasis*), but it works against our need and desire to decrease fat and improve our health (Ladensheim, 2015). Scientific evidence reveals that the body will try to return to its highest lifetime weight; through neurochemical signaling and hormonal changes, the *hypothalamus* slows down energy expenditure and increases appetite to try to adapt to a restrictive calorie diet. These hormonal and neurochemical adaptations can be permanent, making it very difficult for a person with obesity to ever maintain weight in a way that a person who has never been obese can. This might be why obesity tends to be a chronic disease that needs long-term management (Sumithran et al, 2011).

People with obesity often believe, and are subject to, the attitude that obesity is a lifestyle, rather than a disease. The science of obesity has been developing, with new findings coming out every day about the complex interplay among genetics, behavior, mood, environment, the mind, the gut, and neurotransmitters and hormones that keep our energy in and energy out; that is, in—or out of—balance. This opinion, that obesity is a lifestyle issue, is prevalent throughout the general population as well as with many clinicians who haven't had training in obesity management with lifestyle interventions and *pharmacology*. Many people with obesity have a difficult time finding an appropriate and affordable intervention with professional *behaviorists, nutritionists*, and *exercise specialists*, and are left to tackle obesity on their own. The long-term use of medications in other chronic illnesses is well accepted but it is less commonplace with obesity for a variety of reasons. Obesity drugs have a somewhat checkered past, with some removed from the market due to dangerous side effects or the potential for abuse. This leaves many clinicians reluctant to prescribe an anti-obesity medication, especially a newer drug, with limited long-term safety and efficacy data. Their patients might already be on other medications and adding yet another medicine can lead to adverse effects; it might not be clear that the benefits of prescribing outweigh the risks. The medications can be expensive, and insurance is often unwilling to pay for them. From the patient's perspective, the anti-obesity drugs are not always easy to take, and many have side effects. The effectiveness of the medications vary greatly from individual to individual, and moderate weight loss is not always valued or seen as a "success." Also, like use of any long-term medication, it requires surveillance, with the time and expense of visiting their clinician periodically (Cefalu et al, 2015).

Although lifestyle interventions, including diet and exercise, will always form the foundation of weight loss and maintenance, there are six US *Food and Drug Administration* (FDA)–approved medications for the treatment of obesity. These prescription medications can help with the likelihood and the amount of weight lost, beyond what diet and exercise alone can do. These medications include:

For long-term use:

- Liraglutide 3.0 mg (Saxenda)
- Lorcaserin (Belviq)
- Naltrexone/bupropion SR (Contrave)
- Orlistat (Xenical—prescribed; Alli—over-the-counter)
- Phentermine/topiramate (Qsymia)

For short-term use only:

- Phentermine (Lomaira/Adipex)
- Phendimetrazine
- Benzphetamine
- Diethylpropion

How Do These Medications Work?

Each of these medications works in a different way to help you lose weight. Most are small *molecules* that cross the *blood–brain barrier* and activate a *neurochemical* cascade in the brain, with some efficacy toward causing weight loss but also other *central nervous system* (CNS) effects, as well. Newer weight-loss medications are more targeted, mimicking the body's hormones from the gut–brain axis. None are "magic pills," but in conjunction with a healthy diet and regular exercise, they have been shown to result in some degree of weight loss. Most of the medications work by doing the following:

- Reducing your appetite so that you eat fewer calories

- Reducing the absorption of your food, especially fat

- Increasing your energy expenditure, by boosting your metabolism (e.g., by raising your body temperature)

- Mimicking calorie restriction (Chiba et al, 2010).

We briefly review the mechanism of action of each FDA-approved obesity medication.

Long-term medications for obesity:

- *Liraglutide 3.0 mg,* marketed as Saxenda, is an injectable drug that is used to treat diabetes; it was approved in 2015 for weight loss. It slows down the rate of food leaving your stomach, keeps your liver from making too much glucose and helps your pancreas make more insulin, thereby lowering your *blood glucose.* The *glucagon-like peptide* (GLP-1) mimics a hormone that activates a part of your brain that regulates your appetite. It helps you feel less hungry, leading to eating less, and resulting in weight loss (Ladensheim, 2015).

- *Lorcaserin* is sold as Belviq, and it works by selectively activating a type of *serotonin receptor* found in your brain, the 5-HT$_{2c}$ receptor. Triggering the 5-HT$_{2c}$ receptors in the hypothalamus is thought to stimulate the *pro-opiomelanocortin* (POMC) *brain cells* that produce *alpha-melanocyte stimulating hormone* (α–MSH). The α–MSH activates the *melanocortin4 receptors* (MC4R), which induces *satiety,* or a sense that you are not hungry, and might also increase your energy expenditure, burning more calories (http://doi.org/10.1358/dot.2010.46.12.1556433).

- *Naltrexone/bupropion* is the generic name for Contrave, a combination of medications that work in the brain in several ways to help with weight loss. The hypothalamic melanocortin system and the *mesolimbic reward system* regulate food intake and body weight through a *feedback loop.* The POMC brain cells in the hypothalamus release both α–*melanocyte-stimulating hormone* (MSH) and β–*endorphins.* These work in opposite ways to regulate hunger, with the MSH/MC4R decreasing appetite and the β-endorphins encouraging pleasure eating. The α–MSH activates the MC4Rs; the activated MC4Rs decrease your appetite. The POMC cells also release β-endorphins, which are our own natural *opioids* that are activated by "rewards," such as sugary and high-fat foods. The β-endorphins can inactivate the anorectic effect of the MC4Rs through feedback loops, leading to your eating foods that activate the internal opioid system. *Bupropion* is a *dopamine and norepinephrine re-uptake inhibitor* (NDRI), which increases the dopamine and norepinephrine concentrations in the brain. It is hypothesized that hypothalamic dopamine stimulates the POMC MC4R neurons that can decrease food cravings. Bupropion also influences energy expenditure by increasing the body's heat production. Naltrexone is a *μ-opioid antagonist* that prevents β-endorphins from undoing the anorectic effect of the MC4Rs. Naltrexone also prevents an increase in dopamine in the brain's mesolimbic reward system in the *nucleus accumbens*. This prevents the pleasure (i.e., increased dopamine) in reward-eating binges on foods high in sugar and fat. The combination of the two drugs, naltrexone and bupropion, produces a greater reduction in food intake than either drug administered alone (Billes et al, 2014).

- *Orlistat* is marketed as a prescription drug, Xenical, and as an over-the-counter medication as Alli, which is a reduced dose from the prescribed drug. Orlistat is a *pancreatic lipase inhibitor*. It works in the gastrointestinal (GI) tract by binding to lipase, an enzyme produced by the pancreas that breaks down fats. Orlistat reduces lipase's ability to break down triglycerides into components that are normally absorbed. Fats that aren't absorbed leave your body through bowel movements (Lunagariya et al, 2014; Derosa et al, 2016).

- *Phentermine/topiramate ER*, a combination drug prescribed as Qsymia, was the first combination drug approved by the FDA for obesity, in 2012. Phentermine is similar to *amphetamine*, in that it triggers the release of norepinephrine into the neural *synapses* and to a lesser extent, dopamine and *serotonin*. Its main effect is to decrease the sensation of hunger primarily by modulating the effect on the hypothalamus, and it might also increase energy expended to boost metabolism. Topiranate (Topamax) is an anti-seizure drug known to be correlated with weight loss. The mechanism of action of topiramate is unknown, but it is believed to influence the neurotransmitters that regulate appetite and satiety by increasing gamma amino butyric acid (GABA) activity and *carbonic anhydrase inhibition* (Lonneman et al, 2013).

Short-term medications for obesity:

- *Phentermine*, also sold as Adipex, is the most frequently prescribed medication for weight loss. It is a sympathomimetic, similar to amphetamine. It was first approved by the FDA in 1959 and marketed for several years as part of fen-phen, which was taken off the market in 1997 because fenfluramine was found to cause *pulmonary hypertension* and valvular heart disease in a significant number of people taking the drug. Since then, phentermine has been prescribed alone as a *psychostimulant* that increases your heart rate and blood pressure and decreases appetite.

- *Phendimetrazine* is another sympathomimetic that works in your brain to decrease appetite. It is marketed as Bontril and Melfiat.

- *Benzphetamine* is marketed as Didrex and Regimex. It is also a sympathomimetic, similar in action to phentermine. It blunts appetite.

- *Diethylpropion*, prescribed only as a *generic* medication, is also a sympathomimetic, similar in action to phentermine. It blunts appetite.

Off-label prescription medications:

- *Metformin* is a generic diabetes treatment usually sold as Glucophagae which may help people with diabetes or those who have gained weight (e.g., from use of antipsychotics) lose weight. It's mechanism of action is not completely understood, but it is believed to be related to lowering blood glucose, which decreases the *insulin* burden that triggers hunger, leading to a lower calorie intake. It also appears to affect how fat is processed and stored.

- *Topiramate* is a generic anti-seizure drug once used for epilepsy and now more commonly for the prevention of migraines. It has multiple effects on the brain that result in a decreased appetite. It is now often used as part of a combination medication, phentermine and topiramate.

- *Zonisamide* is an anti-seizure drug that has effects on serotonin and dopamine; it also blocks *calcium* and sodium channels. It was identified as causing weight reduction during clinical trials for epilepsy, as an adverse effect. Its exact mechanism of action is unknown, but it appears to alter the sense of taste.

- *Fluoxetine*, also known as Prozac, is a selective serotonin re-uptake inhibitor (SSRI) that can cause weight loss in some individuals (typically those who are underweight or who have an eating disorder). Its mechanism of action is not known, but it can cause a decrease in appetite, nausea (usually only when first started), and dry mouth.

- *Bupropion*, brand named Wellbutrin, is a norepinephrine-dopamine re-uptake inhibitor (NDRI) that works by stimulating the POMC MC4R neurons of the hypothalamus, which can decrease food cravings and increase energy expenditure. It is now marketed as a combination drug along with naltrexone.

What Side Effects Do Anti-Obesity Medications Have?

Each of the anti-obesity medications has side effects, ranging from mild to serious. Several of these medications have been taken off the market due to serious adverse effects; for example, fen-phen in the United States, due to pulmonary hypertension and heart valve damage; rimonabant in the United Kingdom, due to its association with psychiatric disorders, including depression and suicidal tendencies; and *sibutramine* (used from 1997 through 2010, when the Sibutramine Cardiovascular Outcomes [SCOUT] trials showed an association with an increased risk of major cardiovascular events in patients with obesity as compared to those taking placebo). The drugs that have been removed from the market had a different mechanism of action than the medications that are currently FDA approved, so it is not logical to assume that all obesity drugs are dangerous. As always, it is necessary to be informed about the expected benefit of any medication you might consider taking as well as its risks and then determine whether it has a favorable risk–benefit ratio. There is a framework of stepped interventions based on *body mass index* (BMI) and co-morbid health issues to guide clinicians in the selection of treatment for patients with overweight and obesity, based on the guidelines of the National Heart, Lung and Blood Institute (NHLBI) in 1998. This is important because these medications are not used for those with normal BMIs (Bray and Ryan, 2014).

Following are some common and serious adverse medication effects of FDA-approved anti-obesity medications:

Liraglutide 3.0 mg (Saxenda)

Common side effects of liraglutide include nausea, diarrhea, constipation, headache, vomiting, low blood sugar (*hypoglycemia*), decreased appetite, upset stomach, fatigue, dizziness, stomach pain, and changes in enzyme (*lipase*) levels in your blood. There is a *Black Box warning* suggesting that it might induce thyroid cancers.

Lorcaserin (Belviq)

Common reactions include hypoglycemia (low blood sugar), headache, anemia, dizziness, nausea, vomiting, fatigue, *hyperprolactinemia*, diarrhea, dry skin, *bradycardia*, and cognitive impairment. Serious reactions include the risk of *serotonin syndrome*, pulmonary hypertension, valvular heart disease risk, bradycardia, and psychiatric disorders (including depression and thoughts of suicide).

Naltrexone/bupropion SR (Contrave)

Common reactions include nausea/vomiting, headaches, dizziness, insomnia, diarrhea, increased blood pressure and heart rate, anxiety, flushing, fatigue, tremor, ringing in the ears, and irritability. Serious adverse effects include neuropsychiatric symptoms, *suicidality*, *Stevens-Johnson syndrome*, severe hypertension, *hepatotoxicity*, and seizures.

Orlistat (Xenical—prescribed; Alli—over-the-counter)

Common reactions to orlistat include oily stool spotting, flatus with discharge, *fecal urgency and incontinence*, fatty stools, an increased number of stools, fatigue, dizziness, and rectal discomfort. Adverse effects that can be severe include fat-soluble vitamin deficiency, hepatotoxicity, *nephrotoxicity*, and *oxalate nephropathy*.

Phentermine/topiramate (Qsymia)

Common side effects include *paresthesias* (a burning or prickling sensation of your hands, feet, or other parts of the body), dry mouth, constipation, a metallic taste, insomnia, dizziness, headache, nausea, back pain, fatigue, diarrhea, blurred vision, depression, anxiety, attention disturbance, and cognitive impairment. Serious reactions can include severe *metabolic acidosis* (a disturbance of the electrolytes in your blood), *kidney stones*, adverse effects on your bones (such as *osteoporosis*), increased body temperature, rapid heart rates, pulmonary hypertension, Stevens-Johnson syndrome, suicidal thinking, and seizure (if stopped abruptly).

For short-term use only (less than 12 weeks):

Phentermine (Lomaira/Adipex)

When first beginning phentermine/topiramate extended release (ER), the dose is titrated up over 14 days to improve its tolerability. Common side effects include *palpitations*, rapid heart rate, elevated blood pressure, restlessness, dizziness, insomnia, a change in mood, tremor, headache, dry mouth, an unpleasant taste, impotence, and a change in *libido*. Serious adverse events include *cardiac ischemia* (i.e., a condition in which the heart does not receive enough blood flow), elevated blood pressures and heart rates, pulmonary hypertension, *psychosis,* symptoms of dependency and withdrawal (if it is abruptly discontinued).

Phendimetrazine, benzphetamine, diethylpropion

Similar common and serious side effects as *phentermine*.

Following are common and serious adverse medication effects of off-label anti-obesity medications:

- *Metformin* has several common side effects, including diarrhea, nausea, vomiting, abnormal weakness or a lack of energy, indigestion, decreased appetite, headache, a metallic taste, and rash. More serious adverse effects include lactic acidosis, *megaloblastic anemia*, and *liver toxicity*.

- *Topiramate* has a long list of possible side effects, including metabolic acidosis, tingling of the extremities, sleepiness, dizziness, fatigue, nervousness, a lack of appetite, cognitive dysfunction, problems with balance, and *ataxia*, mood disturbances, and others. Serious adverse reactions can include severe metabolic acidosis, kidney stones, problems with bones (such as osteoporosis), *hyperammonemic encephalopathy*, psychosis, suicidal thinking, anemias, glaucoma, Stevens-Johnson syndrome, and *withdrawal seizures* (if abruptly discontinued).

- *Zonisamide* can cause sleepiness, dizziness, nausea, headaches, irritability, agitation, fatigue, impaired concentration, impaired memory, confusion, depression, insomnia, double vision, speech disturbance, and diarrhea. Serious reactions include Stevens-Johnson syndrome, changes in your blood (e.g., *aplastic anemia*), *hyperthermia* and *heat stroke*, *pancreatitis*, depression, suicidality, psychosis, rhabdomyolosis, status epilepticus, and withdrawal seizures if abruptly discontinued.

- *Fluoxetine* can cause insomnia, nervousness, nausea, headache, diarrhea, dry mouth, a decrease in libido, yawing, tremor, dizziness, and sweating. Serious reactions can include suicidal thinking, *hypomania/mania*, heart rhythm problems (such as torsades de pointes), serotonin syndrome, *hyponatremia,* and other adverse effects.

- *Bupropion* commonly causes a dry mouth, headache, agitation, nausea, and dizziness. Some might experience tremor, sweating, abnormal dreams, insomnia, and ringing in the ears. Serious reactions include suicidal thinking, mania, *homicidal ideation*, seizures, severe hypertension, *myocardial infarction*, *arrhythmias*, Stevens-Johnson syndrome, and hepatotoxicity.

What Over-The-Counter Weight-Loss Medications Are Available and Should I Use Them?

For many reasons, only a small percentage of people with obesity who could benefit from prescribed medications to enhance weight loss ever receives a prescription. As noted earlier, this can be from a number of causes, including worry about side effects, a lack of knowledge of available options, the financial burden of expensive medications and surveillance, and the time it takes and sometimes the embarrassment of talking to a physician about treatment options. There is also a growing interest in *complementary and alternative medicine* (CAM). A quick search of the internet or a drug store aisle quickly reveals numerous "magic pills" available for purchase. This offers privacy and generally a lower price point to start treatment, but there are some very serious things to consider before beginning your own "natural" treatments.

Diet supplements, vitamins, minerals, herbal remedies, and *nutraceuticals* are considered dietary supplements and are not FDA approved. Therefore, the industry is largely unregulated and can make claims without scientific studies to back up their claims. The purity of the ingredients can be questionable, and it is possible that not all ingredients are listed accurately. Caffeine is sometimes added to increase the stimulant effect. One study found that 47% of the samples analyzed contained more than 400 mg of caffeine, above the safe limit; excess amounts of caffeine can lower your seizure threshold, cause palpitations, and increase your blood pressure (Neves and Caldas, 2017). The dose of the supplement is not necessarily correct, particularly given that there are seldom any quality clinical trials done to determine dose and efficacy.

"Natural" does not equal "safe." Many of the herbs and nutraceuticals have very significant side effects on the heart and liver or can have interactions with medications you are currently taking. A common "natural" product we sometimes use is grapefruit juice, which can interfere with other medications, especially *cholesterol* and drugs to lower your blood pressure, which could lead to severe adverse effects. It is very important to discuss any supplement you are thinking about taking with your health-care provider. You can also do some research on your own via the internet at the National Center for Complementary and Integrative Health (https://nccih.nih.gov/). This is a government organization that provides unbiased information on alternative and complementary non-prescription medications, including reviews of clinical trials and safety information.

The *American Association of Clinical Endocrinologists* established medical guidelines for the clinical use of dietary supplements and nutraceuticals in 2003. Many studies of alternative dietary supplements and nutriceuticals (DS/N) were reviewed, and none were found to have demonstrated safety and efficacy by more than one peer-reviewed study. This is its statement:

> "Because the principle of 'do no harm' cannot be guaranteed in light of (1) the multiplicity and complexity of DS/N-food-medication interactions and (2) the lack of sufficient scientific substantiation to outweigh potential risks, AACE cannot recommend the use of any DS/N or nonprescription product for obesity management (grade D)." (https://doi.org/10.4158/EP.9.5.417)

Likewise, we cannot recommend any over-the-counter supplement for weight loss. Many have drug-like effects that are unpredictable and could be dangerous. Some are toxic in larger doses, and most have not been well studied. Here, we have chosen a few of the many dietary supplements on the market and discuss the purported benefits and known risks.

- *Garcinia cambogia* is hydroxycitric acid that is extracted from dehydrated fruit rind, commonly used in cooking in Southern India. It works by preventing the activity of an enzyme in the body that lessens appetite. There are no side effects, based on the fact that it has been taken for centuries. Studies show a modest effect on weight loss in humans in short trials; that is, more than 12 weeks.

- *Camellia sinensis* is a green tea produced from the *C. sinensis* plant that contains polyphenols that influence the *sympathetic nervous system*. This increases energy expenditure, which is the only effect that has been proven in studies to affect weight. There is very little evidence that is suppresses appetite.

- *Chromium picolinate* is thought to boost glucose metabolism and affect the neurotransmitters that regulate food cravings and eating behaviors. There is not enough evidence found in a recent review (Esteghamati et al, 2015) to verify any claims of efficacy or safety of this product.

- *Hoodia gordonii* is one of the most popular "natural" weight-loss products. It has been used in South Africa by the bushmen of the Kalahari Desert traditionally to suppress thirst and hunger during hunts. It was initially investigated by the South Africa Council for Scientific and Industrial Research, which licensed an agreement with a British pharmaceutical company, PhytoPharm, which then collaborated with Pfizer to study the extract. Pfizer ended its collaboration in 2003 due to difficulty with synthesizing the extract into a drug. Unilever then collaborated with PhytoPharm, but it ended the collaboration in 2008 saying that the extract could not meet expectations for safety and efficacy. There are very few scientific studies on Hoodia; nevertheless, it enjoys robust sales to unwary consumers (Misra, 2013).

- Other over-the-counter products on the market are Hydroxycut, which contains caffeine and some herbs, caffeine, Raspberry Ketones, Green Coffee Bean Extract, Glucomannan, Meratrim, Green Tea Extract, Conjugated Linoleic Acid (CLA), Forskolin, Bitter Orange/Synephrine, Meltdown, One XS, F.A.S. Lean, Xtreme Lean, and numerous others. Most of these products have little or no safety or efficacy data for short- or long-term use, and they are not regulated by the FDA.

The quest for safe and effective medications to treat the chronic disease of obesity is an ongoing search. We now have several options to choose from, including medications that can be used long term, with at least some safety data. As we learn more about the complex signaling and feedback loops in our bodies, researchers can create other drugs that target some of the factors that lead to obesity. A healthy lifestyle will always be an essential part of any treatment of obesity. However, for some people with obesity, adding a medication to their regimen might help them achieve and maintain the health benefits of weight loss.

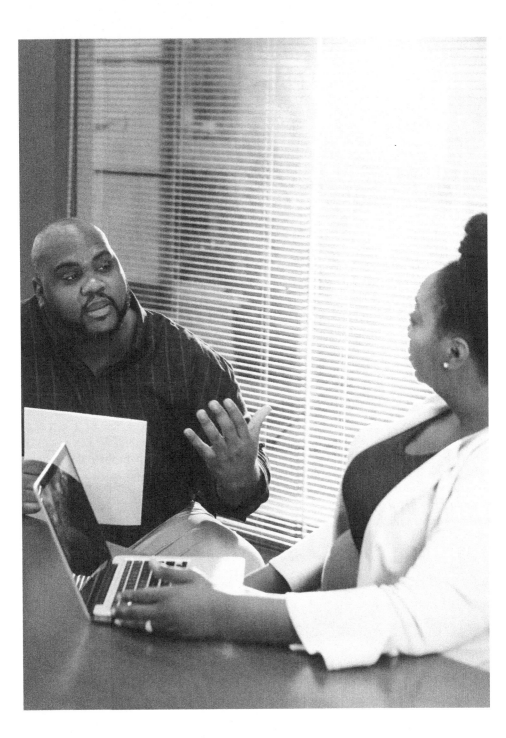

WHAT TYPES OF WEIGHT-LOSS SURGERY OR WEIGHT PROCEDURES ARE AVAILABLE?

Juliana Simonetti, MD

CHAPTER

In This Chapter

- What Is Weight-Loss (Bariatric) Surgery?

- Is Weight-Loss Surgery for Me?

- Am I a Suitable Candidate for Weight-Loss Surgery?

- Why Does My Body Mass Index Matter?

- Why Do I Have to Go Through a Screening for Different Bariatric-Surgery Programs?

- Are There Any Weight-Loss Requirements Before Bariatric Surgery?

- What Types of Weight-Loss Surgery Are Available?

What Is Weight-Loss (Bariatric) Surgery?

Weight-loss surgery has been proven to offer long-lasting effects for weight loss for those with moderate to severe obesity. Contrary to what many might say, weight-loss surgery is not the easy way out. It requires a life-long commitment to diet, exercise, and medical care. Given the commitment required to benefit from surgery, it is essential to understand all available surgical options as you embark on this journey.

Weight-loss surgery, also called *bariatric surgery*, includes several operations that change the digestion of food and the absorption of nutrients by making the stomach smaller and at times by rerouting the intestine, which leads to a significant and lasting amount of weight loss over time. Several studies have shown that bariatric surgery increases life expectancy and decreases the risk of death from *diabetes* by 92%, from cancer by 60%, and from *coronary artery disease* and *heart attacks* by 56% as compared to those with obesity who do not have surgery (Sjöström et al, 2007). In addition, over the past 60 years since it was first performed, bariatric surgery has become much safer. As per the United States Agency of Healthcare Research and Quality (AHRQ), the risk of death from bariatric surgery is now about 0.1% (1 of every 1,000 patients) which is considerably lower than the risk of death from other common surgeries (such as gallbladder removal); the overall probability of having a major complication from bariatric surgery is about 4% (AHRQ, 2007). This decrease in risk can be attributed to technological advancements in the use of minimally invasive techniques. Today, most bariatric surgeries are done *laparoscopically*. This means that the surgery is performed by making very small surgical incisions in the abdomen (with surgeons using special tools to see and work inside the body). The minimally invasive technique allows for faster recovery, shorter hospital stays, less pain, and a lower risk of complications.

Is Weight-Loss Surgery for Me?

By the time someone makes the decision to go forward with surgery, they have typically made many attempts to lose weight and have either not lost the amount of weight that they expected, or they regained the weight they had lost. There can be self-blame or shame for "lack of self-control or will-power"; however, our genetics, human evolution, and the environment each play a significant role in making it easy to gain and to maintain weight and extremely difficult to lose weight. These mechanisms function like a spring: As soon as we lose a certain amount of weight our bodies release *hormones* to make us feel hungrier, increase our cravings for higher caloric foods, and decrease our metabolism. This pulls our weight back to its baseline, where it was previously. This regulation of our bodies' metabolism at a higher weight is called the *set point*, and some of the weight-loss surgeries (such as the *vertical sleeve gastrectomy*, *Roux-en-Y gastric bypass*, and *distal gastric bypass*) can help reset our metabolism and overcome this set point (Müller et al, 2010).

There is more to weight-loss surgery than just decreasing the size of the stomach caus-ing someone to eat less; removing part of the stomach changes the communication between the gut and the brain, affecting hunger and *satiety* (the sensation of feeling full). This hap-pens via a complex mechanism of hormones that are released from the stomach and the intestines and then sensed by the brain leading to a decreased sensation of hunger and improving satiety even when eating smaller amounts of food. In addition, these surgeries induce changes in hormones released by the stomach and intestine to help better metabo-lize sugars. These changes often lead to improvement in diabetes shortly after surgery, even before significant weight loss is achieved. Other benefits of weight-loss surgery include improvements of multiple serious medical conditions such as *hypertension, obstructive sleep apnea*, and *high cholesterol*. In addition, quality of life can markedly improve.

Am I a Suitable Candidate for Weight-Loss Surgery?

The *National Institute of Health* (NIH) has created clinical guidelines with specific criteria about who should have surgery in the United States. Bariatric surgery is available for those with obesity, meaning a body mass index greater than or equal to 40 or a body mass index greater than or equal to 35 with diagnosis of *type 2 diabetes*, or two other medical problems associated with having overweight or obesity with the most commonly approved diseases of heart disease and obstructive sleep apnea. But there can also be consideration for diseases, such as hypertension, high cholesterol, arthritis, and non-alcoholic fatty liver (NAFLD) (Gastrointestinal Surgery for Severe Obesity. NIH Consensus Statement Online, 1991) who have had unsuccessful attempts to lose weight.

Why Does My Body Mass Index Matter?

Body mass index (BMI) is a more accurate calculation of body size and fat than is weight alone. It is often used as a tool to help health-care providers assess the risk of developing certain diseases related to having overweight or obesity, and to help decide who qualifies for bariatric surgery. However, this is only one aspect of a very complex equation used in the assessment of who is a good candidate for surgery. BMI can be calculated by using the following equation:

BMI = weight in pounds (____) × 703/height in inches squared (_____).

Or an easier way is to use the online calculator at the NIH site (https://www.nhlbi.nih.gov/health/educational/lose_wt/BMI/bmicalc.htm).

Or, download the free "NIH BMI" APP on your smart phone.

You can also look at your height and weight in a BMI chart, as shown in Figure 12-1. For example, for someone who is 5 feet 6 inches (66 inches) and has a weight of 223 lbs, their BMI is 36.

Height (inches)	Normal						Overweight					Obese										Extreme Obesity														
BMI	19	20	21	22	23	24	25	26	27	28	29	30	31	32	33	34	35	36	37	38	39	40	41	42	43	44	45	46	47	48	49	50	51	52	53	54
												Body Weight (pounds)																								
58	91	96	100	105	110	115	119	124	129	134	138	143	148	153	158	162	167	172	177	181	186	191	196	201	205	210	215	220	224	229	234	239	244	248	253	258
59	94	99	104	109	114	119	124	128	133	138	143	148	153	158	163	168	173	178	183	188	193	198	203	208	212	217	222	227	232	237	242	247	252	257	262	267
60	97	102	107	112	118	123	128	133	138	143	148	153	158	163	168	174	179	184	189	194	199	204	209	215	220	225	230	235	240	245	250	255	261	266	271	276
61	100	106	111	116	122	127	132	137	143	148	153	158	164	169	174	180	185	190	195	201	206	211	217	222	227	232	238	243	248	254	259	264	269	275	280	285
62	104	109	115	120	126	131	136	142	147	153	158	164	169	175	180	186	191	196	202	207	213	218	224	229	235	240	246	251	256	262	267	273	278	284	289	295
63	107	113	118	124	130	135	141	146	152	158	163	169	175	180	186	191	197	203	208	214	220	225	231	237	242	248	254	259	265	270	278	282	287	293	299	304
64	110	116	122	128	134	140	145	151	157	163	169	174	180	186	192	197	204	209	215	221	227	232	238	244	250	256	262	267	273	279	285	291	296	302	308	314
65	114	120	126	132	138	144	150	156	162	168	174	180	186	192	198	204	210	216	222	228	234	240	246	252	258	264	270	276	282	288	294	300	306	312	318	324
66	118	124	130	136	142	148	155	161	167	173	179	186	192	198	204	210	216	223	229	235	241	247	253	260	266	272	278	284	291	297	303	309	315	322	328	334
67	121	127	134	140	146	153	159	166	172	178	185	191	198	204	211	217	223	230	236	242	249	255	261	268	274	280	287	293	299	306	312	319	325	331	338	344
68	125	131	138	144	151	158	164	171	177	184	190	197	203	210	216	223	230	236	243	249	256	262	269	276	282	289	295	302	308	315	322	328	335	341	348	354
69	128	135	142	149	155	162	169	176	182	189	196	203	209	216	223	230	236	243	250	257	263	270	277	284	291	297	304	311	318	324	331	338	345	351	358	365
70	132	139	146	153	160	167	174	181	188	195	202	209	216	222	229	236	243	250	257	264	271	278	285	292	299	306	313	320	327	334	341	348	355	362	369	376
71	136	143	150	157	165	172	179	186	193	200	208	215	222	229	236	243	250	257	265	272	279	286	293	301	308	315	322	329	338	343	351	358	365	372	379	386
72	140	147	154	162	169	177	184	191	199	206	213	221	228	235	242	250	258	265	272	279	287	294	302	309	316	324	331	338	346	353	361	368	375	383	390	397
73	144	151	159	166	174	182	189	197	204	212	219	227	235	242	250	257	265	272	280	288	295	302	310	318	325	333	340	348	355	363	371	378	386	393	401	408
74	148	155	163	171	179	186	194	202	210	218	225	233	241	249	256	264	272	280	287	295	303	311	319	326	334	342	350	358	365	373	381	389	396	404	412	420
75	152	160	168	176	184	192	200	208	216	224	232	240	248	256	264	272	279	287	295	303	311	319	327	335	343	351	359	367	375	383	391	399	407	415	423	431
76	156	164	172	180	189	197	205	213	221	230	238	246	254	263	271	279	287	295	304	312	320	328	336	344	353	361	369	377	385	394	402	410	418	426	435	443

Figure 12-1: BMI chart. (Source: nhlbi.nih.gov)

Why Do I Have to Go Through a Screening for Different Bariatric-Surgery Programs?

Most bariatric surgical programs have their own criteria for approving patients for bariatric surgery. Although these steps can delay the process or be merely a bureaucratic step, they have been developed to assure patients' safety; they are extremely important for weight-loss surgery candidates. Most programs follow the national recommendations for bariatric surgery and screen patients for contraindications for bariatric surgery as well as their readiness for this life-altering procedure. Patients are typically evaluated by a *registered dietician* who works with patients to change their eating habits while preparing them for post-operative dietary adjustments and nutritional requirements, such as appropriate amounts of proteins and fluids. Dietitians will also educate patients about the use of post-op vitamins and the requirements for mineral supplements. Most programs require a few visits with a dietitian, who is likely to become the patient's best ally through the weight-loss journey during the *pre-operative* and *post-operative* phases.

Are There Any Weight-Loss Requirements Before Bariatric Surgery?

Health insurance companies often require that patients lose weight before being approved for bariatric surgery. Most will aim for 5% to 10% (so for someone who weighs 250 lbs., around 12.5 to 25 lbs. must be lost before having surgery). Although multiple studies have shown inconclusive results regarding the long-term benefits of pre-operative weight loss, some have shown that for those who lose more than 5% of their weight before undergoing a laparoscopic Roux-en-Y gastric bypass, the risk of surgical complication decreases by 13% (Anderin et al, 2015), and it can decrease the length of hospital stay post-operation (Van Nieuwenhove et al, 2011; Giordano and Victorzon, 2014). Some bariatric surgery programs have different preoperative weight-loss requirements.

Psychological Evaluation

Most bariatric surgical programs require a *psychological evaluation* prior to being approved for bariatric surgery. This is done as a safety measure, given that there are some behavioral and psychiatric conditions (e.g., depression, substance abuse, and binge eating) that can have an adverse effect on postoperative recovery and success (Fabricatore et al, 2006). Although most patients view bariatric surgery as a positive event with many psychological benefits, there is a small subset of patients with depression who might develop more depressive symptoms following bariatric surgery. There is also an increase in the number of suicides after bariatric surgery (Omalu et al, 2007). Some reports have suggested that this worsening depression might be due to the added stress of surgery and possibly difficulty taking anti-depressant medications in the post-operative period (Kodama et al, 1998). In addition, there is an increased risk of substance (especially alcohol) abuse (King et al, 2018). Reasons for this include psychological and physiological changes after weight-loss surgery. Addiction transfer (when one trades their "addiction for food" to an addiction to drugs and alcohol) can occur (McFadden, 2010). Another possible reason is that after bariatric procedures (such as gastric bypass surgery), alcohol absorption and sensitivity can heighten its affect in the body. Studies have also suggested that patients who have had problems with binge eating tend to lose less weight and to re-gain more weight after surgery (Rowston et al, 1992).

Given the potential risk posed to some individuals with associated behavioral and psychological conditions, the NIH established pre-operative psychiatric evaluation recommendations (Gastrointestinal Surgery for Severe Obesity. NIH Consensus Statement Online 1991). These recommendations help bariatric surgical teams determine a patient's safety and readiness for surgery. This evaluation is often completed by a *psychologist* who assesses multiple aspects of a patient's life; for example, their support system, living conditions, understanding of the surgery, expectations regarding surgical results, ability to adhere to medical recommendations, eating-related behaviors (prior weight-loss attempts, diet, exercise), and psychiatric conditions such as depression and substance abuse (Flores et al, 2014).

Even if someone has one of the aforementioned problems, it is important to remember that medical and behavioral health treatments are available. Often, when someone is followed by a member of the behavioral health team (and these problems are well controlled), the individual might qualify for bariatric surgery.

Medical Evaluation

A medical evaluation helps to determine whether you are healthy enough for weight-loss surgery and decide what would be the best procedure to perform. In addition, many tests are performed to assess whether there are obesity-related diseases (e.g., *obstructive sleep apnea, diabetes, high blood pressure, high cholesterol*) that can be better managed before surgery to decrease your surgical risk and to improve your outcome.

Some of the pre-bariatric surgical tests that are required include the following:

- Blood work: *complete blood count* (CBC), *kidney function tests* (creatine and blood urea nitrogen), *electrolytes, thyroid-stimulating hormone* (TSH), *liver function tests* (ALT/AST), cholesterol levels, *Helicobacter pylori* (*H. pylori*) antibody (this is a common bacterial infection in the stomach that can pre-dispose you to gastric ulcers), iron levels, vitamin levels (vitamin D, vitamin B_{12}, thiamine)

- Urine analyses

- *Electrocardiogram* (EKG)

- Abdominal *ultrasound* (US)

- Upper-gastrointestinal evaluation (either by *endoscopy* or by drinking a contrast fluid and having an *X-ray*)

- *Pulmonary function tests* (if you have a history of lung problems such as asthma or a history of smoking)

- Sleep study

- *Echocardiogram* and *cardiac stress test* (if you have a history of heart attack or heart problems)

- Medical clearance

Contraindications to Bariatric Surgery (AAFP 2016: Obesity: Indications and Contraindications):

- Bariatric surgery might be contraindicated when the risk of the surgery outweighs its health benefits.

- Pregnancy, or plans to become pregnant within 2 years of surgery, is a contra-indication for surgery. Pregnancy within 2 years of having bariatric surgery can place both you and the baby at significant risk due to changes in the anatomy of the stomach and issues with nutrient absorption. It is important that you plan to avoid pregnancy after surgery because weight loss often enhances fertility.

- Smoking can increase your risk of serious surgical complications. Most bariatric-surgery programs recommend stopping smoking at least 2 months before surgery.

- Ongoing drug and alcohol abuse can affect post-operative healing, increase your risk of ulcers and life-threating nutrient deficiencies as well as worsen addiction and depression.

- *Portal vein hypertension*, often associated with certain liver conditions (such as chronic *hepatitis* and alcoholic *cirrhosis*), can lead to an increase in *portal hypertension* and serves as a contraindication to surgery.

- Advanced cancer.

- Severe psychiatric conditions.

- Untreated eating disorders.

- Significant cognitive impairment that would prevent someone from fully understanding the risks and implications of having bariatric surgery serves as a contraindication to surgery.

In addition, each procedure has its own contraindications. *Laparoscopic adjustable gastric banding* is contraindicated in those who take steroid medications for long periods (e.g., *inflammatory bowel diseases* [*Crohn's disease*, chronic *pancreatitis*]) (AAFP 2016: Obesity: Indications and Contraindications). *Laparoscopic sleeve gastrectomy* is contraindicated for those with *Barrett's esophagus* and severe *gastroesophageal reflux disease* (Gagner, 2016). *Roux-en-Y gastric bypass* and *distal gastric bypass* (*duodenal switch* and *biliopancreatic division*) are relatively contraindicated for those with inflammatory bowel disease (Maloney et al, 2011).

What Types of Weight-Loss Surgery Are Available

Operations that make the stomach smaller are called *restrictive surgeries* because these procedures restrict or limit the amount of food and calories that you can eat (which leads to weight loss). The restrictive procedures include *gastric banding* and the *vertical sleeve gastrectomy*.

Gastric Banding ("Lap-Band")

Gastric banding uses an adjustable silicone band that is placed with minimally invasive surgery around the upper part of the stomach, thereby reducing the size of the stomach. A small *port*, the size of a coin, rests under the skin in the abdomen, and it is attached to the silicone band. The band size can be adjusted after the surgery by injecting fluid into this port. Filling the band with more fluid causes it to further restrict the passage of food and liquids through the rest of the digestive system, decreasing the amount of food you can eat and thereby leading to weight loss (O'Brien et al, 2002).

The lap-band procedure is indicated for those older than 18 years and who have a BMI greater than 40 or a BMI greater than 35 with other diagnoses (e.g., diabetes, hypertension, obstructive sleep apnea) associated with having overweight or obesity. Lap-band surgery is a safe procedure with a low risk of severe side effects and mortality, just 0.02% (AAFP 2016: Obesity: Indications and Contraindications). It causes more gradual weight loss than other bariatric procedures; the average weight loss is 47% of excess body weight (Excess body weight = ideal body weight − current weight) (O'Brien et al, 2013). For a woman (ideal body weight is 100 lbs. for the first 5 feet, plus 5 lbs. for each additional inch; for a man it is 106 lbs. for the first 5 feet, plus 6 lbs. for each additional inch (Peterson et al, 2016).

Although lap-band surgery is safe and can lead to long-term weight loss, it has fallen out of favor in the United States; many surgical centers no longer do this procedure. One reason for this is that it has a higher rate of complications and a more frequent need for re-operation. Some recent studies have noted that almost half of patients who have the lap-band had a follow-up procedure for complications (such as pouch enlargement, erosion, and port and tube problems). Six percent of patients have also had the band removed (O'Brien et al, 2013). Another reason why the lap band has fallen out of favor is because it is not a *metabolic procedure*. This means that it does not change the communication between the brain and the gut, which leads to more sustainable weight loss.

Vertical Sleeve Gastrectomy

The vertical sleeve gastrectomy has become the most common weight-loss surgical procedure in the United States, with more than 100,000 surgeries done each year. This procedure has been found to be safe and effective for long-term effects on weight loss. Studies have shown that patients lose an average of 55% of their excess body weight (i.e., if a patient has 100 pounds of excess weight, they will lose on average 55 lbs.) after having a gastric sleeve placed (*American Society for Metabolic and Bariatric Surgery* [ASMBS] website, *sleeve gastrectomy as bariatric procedure.* https://asmbs.org/resources/sleeve-gastrectomy-as-a-bariatric-procedure. 2012). There is also a significant improvement or resolution of some obesity-related diseases (e.g., obstructive sleep apnea, high blood pressure, high cholesterol, fatty liver, arthritis, infertility, polycystic ovarian syndrome [PCOS]). One study showed that diabetes resolved in two-thirds of patients and improved in approximately one-fourth after 1 year in those who had a sleeve gastrectomy (Gill et al, 2010). In addition, numerous studies have shown improvement in quality of life.

This procedure is typically performed laparoscopically whereby most of the stomach (approximately three-fourths) is removed. The remainder of the stomach is reattached with surgical staples forming a long tube, or "sleeve," leaving a banana-shaped stomach (Shi et al, 2010). This procedure takes roughly 1 to 2 hours in the operating room. The recovery time varies; it often takes 1 to 3 days before you can leave the hospital (Sucandy et al, 2013). Some bariatric programs send patients home on the day of the surgery. Patients can return to work within 1 to 3 weeks depending on their type of work; however, heavy lifting (i.e., more than 10 lbs.) is not allowed for 4 to 6 weeks.

Patients are thought to lose weight via two mechanisms: by decreasing the stomach size and by restricting the amount of food someone can consume. The other mechanism is by decreasing appetite, given that the surgery removes the part of the stomach that produces a hunger hormone, called *ghrelin* (Gumbs et al, 2007). Therefore, patients not only feel full after eating a smaller amount of food, but they also feel less hungry.

The sleeve gastrectomy is a safe procedure; the risk of mortality is 0.2% according to the ASMBS. The risk of post-operative complications is also low (e.g., leakage from the staples in the stomach [2.2%], bleeding [1.2%], and narrowing of the passage of the stomach, called *stricture* [0.6%]). The most commonly reported longer-term complication related to this procedure is gastro-esophageal reflux (manifest by heartburn and regurgitation), which is seen in 21% of patients (Himpens et al, 2010). This complication is often treated with a class of medication called *proton pump inhibitors.* Nutritional deficiencies (thought to be due to the decreased absorption of nutrients and vitamins from the stomach with a smaller stomach pouch and a decrease in food intake) are less commonly seen in those with the sleeve gastrectomy than with gastric bypass surgery. Some of the more common mineral and vitamin deficiencies include deficiency of vitamin B_{12}, vitamin D, folate, iron, calcium, and zinc (Sarkosh et al, 2013). This makes it extremely important to follow-up with the surgical bariatric team at 3, 6, and 12 months after surgery and at least yearly after that. Patients are often unaware that life-long follow-up is essential.

Restrictive and Malabsorptive

Other procedures (such as Roux-en-Y gastric bypass and *distal gastric bypass with duodenal switch*, and *biliopancreatic division*) are a combination of restrictive and malabsorptive procedures. The restrictive aspect of this procedure is accomplished by making the stomach smaller; it restricts or limits the amount of food you can eat at one time. The malabsorptive component is caused by bypassing part of the intestine that affects the absorption of food and nutrients. Therefore, when you eat, a smaller percentage of the food will be absorbed. This in turn leads to a lower intake of food and calories and to a long-term effect on weight loss.

Roux-en-Y Gastric Bypass

Until recently, gastric bypass had been one of the most common weight-loss surgeries in the United States, when it became second in popularity to the sleeve gastrectomy. It remains an excellent option for those looking for long-term and sustained weight loss. One study showed an average excess weight loss of 77.6% at 18 months (i.e., if a patient has 100 lbs. of excess weight, they will lose on average 77.6 lbs). For example, if a woman is 5 feet 5 inches tall and weighs 250 lbs., she is 125 lbs. above her ideal weight (excess body weight = ideal body weight – current weight). Post-gastric bypass, she would lose an average of 98 lbs. (125 lbs. × 0.78) in 18 months; her weight would drop to 152 lbs. and her BMI would decrease from 42 to 25. Like the sleeve gastrectomy, there is significant improvement and or resolution of many obesity-related co-morbidities (e.g., hypertension, high cholesterol, osteoarthritis, diabetes). Some studies have shown that remission or resolution of diabetes was higher in patients who had a gastric bypass as compared to those who had the sleeve (with a diabetes remission rate of 80%) (Li et al, 2013). In addition, several studies have shown improvement in the quality of life for those who had this surgery with a decrease in the mortality rate. Patients are not only living longer, they are living better.

Roux-en-Y gastric bypass as with the sleeve gastrectomy is also commonly performed laparoscopically, with minimally invasive techniques, in which the surgeon makes five to six small cuts in the abdomen and inserts a small camera and tools to remove 60% to 80% of the stomach; what is left of the stomach is made into a small pouch that holds approximately 30 ml (roughly the size of a lemon). The newly formed pouch is then attached to the distant part of the intestine, "bypassing" part of it. The purpose of bypassing part of the intestine is that food will have a shorter distance to travel through the digestive tract and, therefore, will not be fully absorbed (Schauer et al, 2000). This surgery leads to changes in the hunger hormone; cutting part of the stomach decreases the amount of hunger hormone released, causing a decrease in appetite.

As previously discussed, gastric bypass surgery has come a long way from its beginnings as an open surgical procedure (which required prolonged time in the operating room and long hospital stays) to its laparoscopic, minimally invasive approach. This has led to shorter operating times, fewer complications, faster recovery, and safer surgery. The average operating time for the laparoscopic gastric bypass is 1.5 to 3.5 hours and the average patients' hospital stay is 2 to 3 days. Recovery time is like that of the sleeve gastrectomy, for which patients can return to work within 2 to 4 weeks depending on the type of work they do; however, heavy lifting (more than 10 lbs.) is not allowed for 4 to 6 weeks.

The mortality rate for the laparoscopic procedure is also low and like that of the sleeve gastrectomy. One study, involving multiple bariatric centers with 2,458 participants, showed a 30-day post-laparoscopic gastric bypass surgery mortality rate of 0.2%. The mortality rate for open procedures, in which the surgeon opens the abdomen to perform the procedure, increases to 2.1% (Belle et al, 2013). The rates of complications have been slightly higher than with the sleeve gastrectomy, with rates ranging from 1% to 5%. Some of the immediate complications include surgical site leaks, bleeding, *bowel obstruction*, *deep vein thrombosis*, and *pulmonary embolism*. Long-term side effects include nutritional deficits with protein as well as with multiple vitamins and minerals, including iron (20%–49%), vitamin B$_{12}$ (26%–70%), and folate (9%–35%), in addition to calcium and vitamin D (Nandagopal et al, 2010). The reason for the nutritional deficits post–gastric bypass is that the stomach is now very small and part of the intestine has been bypassed, allowing food to travel faster through the digestive tract, preventing the absorption of vitamins and nutrients. Some of these deficiencies can lead to life-threating conditions, and it is imperative that patients take their vitamins after having had weight-loss surgery and continue to follow-up with the surgical team.

Biliopancreatic Diversion with Duodenal Switch

Biliopancreatic diversion with duodenal switch (BPD-DS) is a sleeve gastrectomy combined with a gastric bypass in which a larger portion of the intestine is bypassed. This procedure is also most often performed laparoscopically with minimally invasive techniques in which the surgeon makes small openings in the abdomen through which a camera and tools are inserted to remove 70% to 75% of the stomach, forming a tubular, "banana-shaped" stomach. The newly formed stomach is then attached to the furthest part of the small intestine, bypassing almost three-fourths of the intestine. The part of the intestine that was bypassed is the part that carries some of the digestive enzymes (that help to break-down and absorb protein and fats) from the pancreas. This part of the intestine is reattached to the last portion of the intestine; therefore, after surgery, the patient can digest and absorb some of those nutrients (Ren et al, 2000). The benefit of this procedure over the previous two procedures, is that biliopancreatic diversion can lead to more weight loss while allowing patients to eat near-normal amounts of food. Initially this procedure causes a decrease in food intake, like the sleeve gastrectomy and gastric bypass, given the small size of the stomach; however, over time, patients are able to eat almost normal amounts of food. The contributing factor to the long-term weight loss is that even when someone is eating normal amounts, he or she will absorb only a small amount of these calories because most of the intestine is bypassed. Like both sleeve and the bypass surgeries, this procedure also changes the hormone communication to the brain that effects appetite and sugar metabolism.

Although weight-loss results and resolution of obesity-related co-morbidities are greater with this procedure, BPD-DS is a more complex surgery, leading to longer operating times and to potentially more complications. The average operating time is around 4 hours and the hospital stay is on average 4 days, with rates of complications as high as 62% (Ren et al, 2000) and 37% of patients having complications that require surgery (Sethi et al, 2016). Some of these complications were related to nutritional deficiencies (in particular, of vitamin D), anemias, and changes in the hormone (called parathyroid hormone) that controls bone metabolism. However, with technological advancements, the mortality rate with laparoscopic procedure is now like that of the other two procedures, about 0.1%, and more recent reports have noted a decrease in risk of complications of 3% to 7.4%. Excess weight loss (EWL) was 67.9% at 10 to 15 years after the surgery with a resolution of type 2 diabetes of 87.5% (Bolckman et al, 2016).

This is a technically more difficult surgery, and it is very important that it be done by an experienced surgeon. This procedure is offered only at selected bariatric-surgery sites. As with the other two procedures it is quite important to have close follow-up with the surgical team, to take all vitamins as recommended, and to continue having blood work monitored initially at 3, 6, and 12 months, and at least yearly thereafter.

Endoscopic Options

Endoscopic Intragastric Balloon

Placement of an intragastric balloon is a non-surgical option for those with obesity (i.e., with a BMI of 30 to 40) who have failed to lose weight through diet and exercise. Patients are typically placed under light sedation, and medication is given through a vein to make patients feel sleepy and relaxed while not remembering the procedure. This is done by an *anesthesiologist* who is likely to use the same medications as are used during an *endoscopy* or *colonoscopy*. A biocompatible silicone (silicone made of materials that can be used inside the body) deflated balloon is placed in the stomach via the mouth with the help of an endoscope (a small tube with a camera in the tip), and it is then inflated with a saline solution. These procedures usually take only 20 to 30 minutes and patients return home the same day.

There are currently three types of balloons approved by the US *Food and Drug Administration* (FDA) for the treatment of obesity. The first two were approved by the FDA in 2015 and use a liquid to fill the balloon in the stomach. One is the single balloon called

Orbera, and the other is a dual-balloon system, called *ReShape.* Both balloons are filled with a saline solution in the stomach. The ReShape balloons also have a non-toxic dye, called methylene blue; in case the balloon were to rupture, you would be able to see the blue dye in the urine. A third balloon, which was approved by the FDA in 2016, is called *Obalon,* consists of three balloons filled with air. These balloons are swallowed in a capsule, one at time, over a few weeks. After the capsule is in the stomach, it is inflated with gas via a small tube. The purpose of the balloons is to fill a portion of the stomach, giving the sensation of feeling full, which leads to a decrease in appetite and in food intake, causing weight loss. Studies report weight loss for the intragastric balloons, averaging a 28.7% loss of excess weight at 6 months and of 39.2% at 12 months (Kim et al, 2016). All currently available balloons are safe in the stomach for 6 months and must be removed using a minimally invasive endoscopic procedure with light sedation. The most common side effect noted with the balloons is initial abdominal discomfort; nausea, and vomiting can occur for the first few days after the balloon is inserted and tend to improve. One report looked at patients treated with balloons and found that nausea occurred in 72% of patients with the balloon; more serious side effects, such as ulcer, occurred in 5% of those who had the balloon. However, no serious or fatal complication has been reported in these studies (Zheng et al, 2015). Earlier this year the FDA reported acute *pancreatitis* (inflammation of the pancreas), which can be a very serious health condition, in several patients following insertion of both liquid-filled balloons (Orbera and ReShape) due to compression of the pancreas (which is located behind the stomach) by the balloon. All of the cases required sooner-than-expected removal of the balloon, and four of the patients required hospitalization. The FDA also issued an updated alert to health-care providers with five reports of unanticipated deaths in 2016 of patients who had liquid-filled intragastric balloons, four were reported with Orbera and one was with ReShape. This happened within 1 month after the balloon insertion; however, there is no clear evidence that the patient death was related to the balloon placement (Liquid-filled Intragastric Balloon Systems: Letter to Healthcare Providers Potential Risks. Feb 9, 2017 and Aug 10, 2017. https://www.fda.gov/Safety/MedWatch/SafetyInformation/SafetyAlertsforHumanMedicalProducts/ucm570916.htm).

Intragastric balloons are an effective non-surgical option for weight loss; however, this is currently approved for 6 months only and some studies have shown that the weight-loss results are not long lasting. Patients tend to regain weight following balloon removal (Kim et al, 2016). In addition, the balloons are currently not covered by health insurance and require out-of-pocket costs of approximately $7,000 to $10,000 depending upon where it is done. However, this can be a great tool, especially for those who are not surgical candidates and who might consider using the balloon with other medical treatments.

Long-Term Effects of Bariatric Surgery

Weight Loss and Decrease in Mortality

A common misconception is that most patients who have weight-loss surgery will regain their weight. This is untrue; according to the ASMBS, as many as 50% of patients regain a small portion of their weight loss (just 5%) 2 years or more following surgery. However, long-term studies have demonstrated that most patients who have bariatric surgery maintain their weight loss. The Swedish study is one of the largest and longest-running studies on bariatric surgery with more than 2,000 people who had bariatric surgery and were followed for more than 10 years. This study showed that most of the weight loss occurred within the first 2 years after the surgery: 32% of weight loss was found 2 years after gastric bypass, 25% was noted after vertical-banded gastroplasty, and 20% after gastric banding. Most of the weight loss was maintained and stable at 10 years after surgery, with 25% found for gastric bypass, 16% for vertical-banded gastroplasty, and 14% for gastric banding (Sjostrom et al, 2007). In addition, it found that there were more deaths in the group that didn't have bariatric surgery than those who did. The patients who had bariatric surgery had fewer heart attacks, strokes, and cancer. This indicates that bariatric surgery for severe obesity leads to long-term weight loss and to a decreased risk of death.

Decrease in Incidents and Resolution of Co-Morbidities

In addition, there are other benefits to weight-loss surgery, including a lower occurrence of new diagnoses of diabetes, high blood pressure, and elevated cholesterol among those who had weight-loss surgery. There was also resolution or significant improvement of many obesity-related co-morbidities, such as hypertension (by 34% at 2 years), diabetes (by 68% in 2 years, and 33% with long-term remission and significant reduction of anti-diabetic medications) (https://asmbs.org/resources/long-term-survival-benefit-after-metabolic-and-bariatric-surgery). Other conditions, such as obstructive sleep apnea and fatty liver, were also shown to improve in the bariatric-surgery group. There are also reports of increased mobility and physical activity in the post-bariatric group along with improvement in the measures of quality of life (Sjostrom et al, 2007).

Nutritional Deficiency

One of the main long-term complications of bariatric surgery is nutritional deficiency, mostly related to a decrease in absorption of vitamins and minerals (due to the changes in the size of the stomach and by bypassing parts of the intestine). This can be more severe and significant with procedures that bypass portions of the gastrointestinal (GI) tract where nutrients are absorbed. The most common deficiencies are of vitamin B_{12}, vitamin D, folate, iron, calcium, and zinc (Sarkhosh et al, 2013). There are also issues with the parathyroid hormone which is related to bone metabolism and a possible consequence of vitamin D deficiency or rapid weight loss. Therefore, for most of the aforementioned procedures, you will need to take a multi-vitamin with some additional vitamins and minerals for the rest of your life. It is also extremely important to have follow-up with the bariatric surgical team, with blood work done at 3, 6, and 12 months after the surgery and at least yearly after that.

Dumping Syndrome

This is a potential side effect of procedures (such as the gastric bypass and BPD-DS) that bypass portions of the GI tract where nutrients are absorbed. This occurs only in some patients, and it is due to foods high in sugar or fat entering the end of the small intestine at a rapid rate. The reason these foods enter the last part of the intestine quickly is because with these surgeries part of the intestine is bypassed. This causes an immediate release of hormones and symptoms shortly after eating foods high in fat or sugar. These symptoms include dizziness, palpitations, sweating, nausea, vomiting, abdominal cramps, and diarrhea.

Alcohol Intake

Several studies have shown that patients who have had bariatric surgery are more likely to develop an alcohol use disorder (AUD) or suffer a relapse, especially after gastric bypass. This is likely to be due to altered alcohol metabolism due to changes in the anatomy of the stomach and intestine, which causes accelerated alcohol absorption (https://asmbs.org/resources/long-term-survival-benefit-after-metabolic-and-bariatric-surgery). This means that even smaller amounts of alcohol intake could cause someone to become intoxicated. In addition, liquid calories are easily absorbed and can lead to weight gain. Therefore, alcohol is not recommended after bariatric surgery.

Excess Skin

The amount of excess skin after bariatric surgery depends on how long your skin has been stretched, the amount of your weight loss, and your age. It doesn't matter whether the weight is lost quickly or slowly, the elasticity of the skin is dependent on how long the skin has been stretched.

Weight Regain or Inadequate Weight Loss

Although many patients can maintain some weight loss after surgery, others struggle with either inadequate weight loss or weight regain. In these situations, some people undergo revision surgery, but these procedures are often unsuccessful unless there are anatomic issues associated with the initial procedure. For others, they might achieve weight loss with the use of medications in conjunction with lifestyle changes.

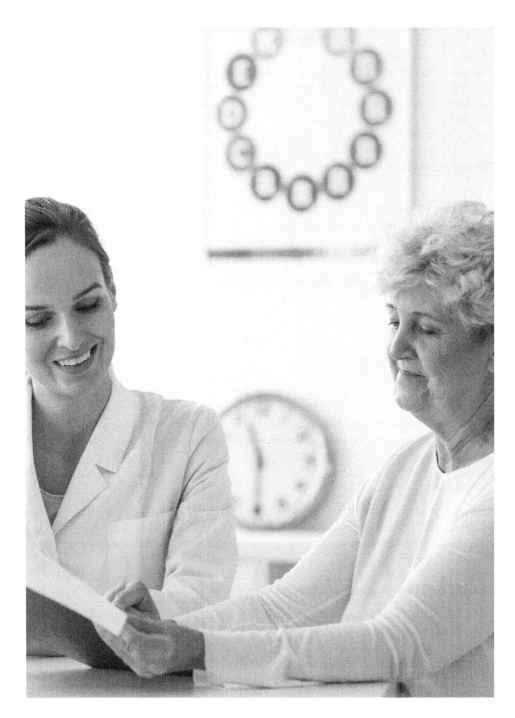

WHAT MIGHT BE THE FUTURE OF OBESITY TREATMENT?

Alexander T. Toth, BA

CHAPTER 13

In This Chapter

- What Is a Clinical Trial and Why Do Such Trials Exist?

- What Types of Clinical Trials Are Being Conducted to Assess Weight Loss?

- What Are the Phases of Clinical Trials?

- What Are the Potential Benefits and Risks of Participating in a Clinical Trial?

- Who Is Eligible for a Clinical Trial?

- Why Should I Enroll in a Clinical Trial?

- What Is Informed Consent?

- What Is a Placebo and Could I Receive It?

- Where Are Clinical Trials Conducted?

- Who Pays for the Cost of a Clinical Trial?

- What Questions Should I Ask Before Joining a Clinical Trial?

- What Happens When a Clinical Trial Is Complete?

What Is a Clinical Trial and Why Do Such Trials Exist?

As increasing numbers of people suffer from obesity and health conditions related to it, it is necessary for medical professionals and scientists to continue to improve current treatments and to develop new treatments for obesity (Cefalu et al, 2015; NIH, 2017a; NIH, 2017b).

To tackle this challenge, the medical community relies on a research process that ensures that the best ideas and treatments make their way into practice. The medical community uses the knowledge and experience to pioneer new treatments and to improve patients' health and quality of life. New ideas are called *hypotheses*; if it is one idea it is called a *hypothesis*. A hypothesis is an idea that medical professionals and scientists believe to be true based on their knowledge. It can be thought of as a well-thought-out educated guess that can be tested to determine whether the hypothesis is correct (e.g., by designing and carrying out carefully planned experiments called *clinical research trials*). A clinical research trial is a research study that evaluates new ways to prevent, detect, or treat disease using a drug or therapy (NIH, 2017b). Clinical trials are particularly important to the future of obesity treatment because they are considered the best type of study for establishing a cause-and-effect relationship; therefore, they are the best way to prove that new drugs or treatments for obesity are effective. Clinical trials offer participants the opportunity to gain access to new treatments (e.g., medications, treatment strategies) that might benefit the participants by helping them to lose weight or improve their health in other ways. It is important to note that clinical trials can also expose participants to certain risks. As a result, clinical trials take place in phases.

What Types of Clinical Trials Are Being Conducted to Assess Weight Loss?

Many clinical trials are being conducted on lifestyle modification (NIH, 2017b), *pharmacotherapy* (drug treatment) (Hassan et al, 2016) (Butsch, 2015), and weight-loss surgery (Gadde & Pritham Raj, 2017). In addition, clinical trials are evaluating the optimal combinations of these treatment modalities (Roslin et al, 2015). Moreover, there are many clinical trials in progress or being proposed for weight loss. These include, but are not limited to, clinical trials that influence the bacteria inside the digestive track and that influence brain pathways through brain stimulation; these studies hope to increase our understanding of how we can use genes to tailor weight-loss treatments (Bof et al, 2017; Corella & Ordovas, 2013; Epstein & Wrotniak, 2010).

What Are the Phases of Clinical Trials?

There are different phases of clinical trials. The first phase of a clinical trial contains the smallest number of people and then builds up to the final phase, which contains the largest number of participants. Studies are run in phases so that different questions can be answered during each phase (Gobe et al, 2017).

- *Phase I trials* comprise about 20 to 80 people and are used to test an experimental drug or treatment for the first time to evaluate its safety and to see whether there are any side effects.

- *Phase II trials* comprise about 100 to 300 people and are used to test the effectiveness of an experimental drug or treatment and to continue to test its safety.

- *Phase III trials* comprise about 1,000 to 3,000 people and are used to confirm the effectiveness of a drug or treatment. It is conducted to look for side effects and to evaluate the drug or treatment in comparison to standard treatment or to similar treatments. This size trial is also used to collect data to determine how to use the drug or the treatment safely.

- *Phase IV trials* are conducted after a drug or treatment has received US *Food and Drug Administration* (FDA) approval and has become available to the public. The drug or treatment's optimal use, safety, and benefits continue to be evaluated in this phase.

What Are the Potential Benefits and Risks of Participating in a Clinical Trial?

Potential Benefits

Clinical trials allow participants to do the following:

- Gain access to new drugs or treatments before they are available to the public

- Provide regular monitoring by doctors and other medical professionals

- Allow patients to make decisions about their health care based on their decision to enroll or not

- Provide an opportunity for participants to help others by furthering medical knowledge (NIH, 2017b)

Potential Risks

Clinical trials can expose participants to the following:

- Clinical trials can involve interventions that cause side effects (that are generally mild and temporary but can be unpleasant). However, even with routine medical care as well as with day-to-day life, serious side effects can occur; fortunately, the chances of this happening are rare.

- Studies might require a longer time commitment and other burdens that might include, but are not limited to, more treatments, more time in a hospital, more blood work, and detailed dosing of experimental medications.

Who Is Eligible for a Clinical Trial?

Clinical trials for obesity and related illnesses enroll both patient volunteers and healthy volunteers. Patient volunteers have obesity and/or a related medical condition, whereas healthy volunteers have neither obesity nor a related illness. Healthy volunteers are included in some clinical trials to serve as a comparison and are often selected based on another similar characteristic (e.g., age, gender) to participants in the study (NIH, 2017b).

Clinical trials for obesity drugs might vary in who they can enroll based on different *inclusion and exclusion criteria* that are based on a variety of factors (e.g., age, gender, disease status, treatment history).

Inclusion criteria are characteristics of participants that *must be true* for them be included in a clinical trial. For example, if the inclusion criteria for a clinical trial include being older than 18 years of age, all participants in that clinical trial would need to be older than the age of 18 years. For a trial on obesity, a study might want to enroll only individuals who have obesity (classified as a *body mass index* [BMI] equal to or greater than 30).

Exclusion criteria are characteristics of participants that *must not be true* for them to become study participants. For example, if the exclusion criteria for a clinical trial wanted to exclude patients younger than 18 years of age, all participants in that clinical trial would need to be 18 years or older. For a trial on obesity, a study might exclude individuals who do not have obesity (i.e., having a BMI equal to or greater than 30).

Why Should I Enroll in a Clinical Trial?

You should enroll in a clinical trial if you think participation in the clinical trial will be of benefit to your health or will benefit you in some other way and if these benefits outweigh any risks that might be involved with the clinical trial. Participants and/or their guardians need to make this decision freely, but the study staff has a duty to fully explain clinical trials and what they entail so that you can make an informed decision (NIH, 2017b).

What Is Informed Consent?

Potential participants in research studies must be given all of the key facts about a clinical trial before they decide whether to participate. *Informed consent* is a process in which potential participants are given the relevant information about the study so that they can decide on their involvement. This process should be ongoing throughout the study. A key component of the informed consent process occurs at the beginning of the study when participants read, sign, and are given a copy of a document called the *consent document*. This document details all relevant information about the study, including the risks and benefits of the study. Signing the document is not a binding agreement to participate in the study, and participants can leave the study at any time and can refuse drugs or treatment at any point.

What Is a Placebo and Could I Receive It?

Although most trials compare a new drug or treatment to another available drug or treatment, some clinical trials administer an inactive drug or treatment that resembles the test drug or treatment during a part of the study. This inactive drug or treatment is called a *placebo*. Placebos are used because they are the most effective way to show that a new drug or treatment has a therapeutic effect (by comparing the results of the placebo group with those of the experimental drug or process). Placebos are not used if their use would put a participant at risk, and you will be told before the study about whether you could receive a placebo. Depending on the study design, you and the study staff might not know during the study whether you are receiving the actual test drug or treatment. This process is called *blinding* and is done to keep the knowledge of which drug or therapy participants are receiving from influencing their outcomes.

Where Are Clinical Trials Conducted?

Clinical trials might be conducted in a variety of settings, including hospitals, doctors' offices, universities, and community clinics. The location often depends on who is conducting the research study.

Who Pays for a Clinical Trial?

Sponsors pay for some or all of the costs of clinical trials. Sponsors might be an organization or an individual, and they can include medical institutions, federal agencies, physicians, voluntary groups, and/or pharmaceutical companies. Some costs of a clinical trial might be billed to participants' insurance companies, if these expenses are part of their normal care, and some expenses might be billed to individuals, depending on the study. You can find information on who is paying for the trial in the consent document.

What Questions Should I Ask Before Joining a Clinical Trial?

All participants should feel comfortable asking the study team any questions they might have before joining a research study. Some additional questions modeled after the US *National Institutes of Health* (NIH) suggested questions are included here, as well, and many of the answers to these questions can be found in the consent document (see Table 13-1).

Table 13-1: Frequently Asked Questions About Clinical Research Trials

What is being studied?
Why do researchers believe the drug or treatment being tested might be effective?
Why might the drug or treatment not be effective?
Has the drug or treatment been tested before?
What are the possible drugs or treatments that I might receive during the trial?
How will it be determined which drugs or treatments I receive?
Who will know which drug or treatment I receive during the trial? Will I know? Will members of the research team know?
How do the possible risks, side effects, and benefits of this trial compare with those of my current treatment?
What will I have to do?
What tests and procedures are involved?
How often will I have to visit the hospital or clinic?
Will hospitalization be required?
How long will the study last?
Who will pay for my participation?
Will I be reimbursed for other expenses?
What type of long-term follow-up care is part of this trial?
If I benefit from the drug or treatment, will I be allowed to continue receiving it after the trial ends?
Will results of the study be provided to me?
Who will oversee my medical care while I am participating in the trial?
What are my options if I am injured during the study?

What Happens When a Clinical Trial Is Complete?

After a clinical trial has been completed, the study staff does a careful analysis of the data they collected to determine the meaning of that data and what future testing they might choose to conduct.

The phase of the trial dictates what happens after a clinical trial:

- After a Phase I or Phase II trial, the data collected is used to decide whether to move on to the next phase of trials, based on whether the drug or treatment is safe or effective.

- After a Phase III trial, the data is analyzed to decide whether the results have medical importance.

The results from clinical trials are generally published in *peer-reviewed scientific journals*. Peer review is a process in which experts in the field review the data, the analysis, and the conclusions that are drawn from the trial before the results are published to make sure that the research is valid. Sometimes, results are discussed at scientific conferences, among the medical community, and in the media if they are of importance to the general public. If a new drug or treatment is proven to be safe and effective in a clinical trial, it might go on to become a part of standard care for a disease or condition.

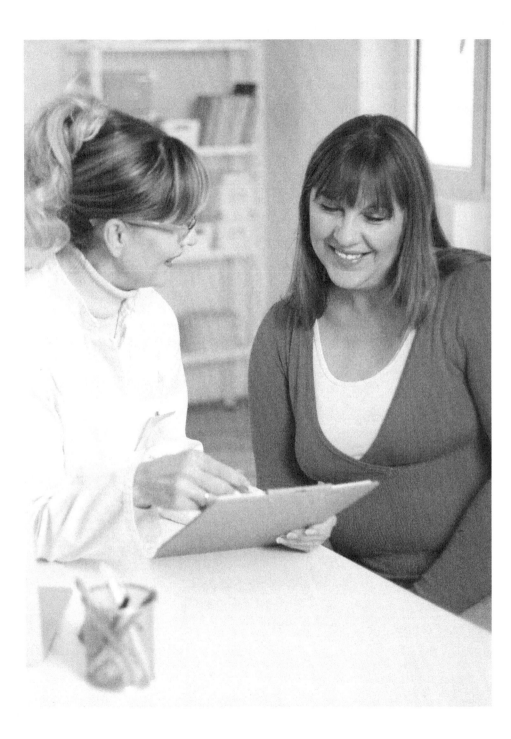

WHICH TYPES OF PROVIDERS CAN HELP ME WITH MY OBESITY?

Tiffani Bell Washington, MD

CHAPTER 14

In This Chapter

- Is Multi-Disciplinary Care Right for Me?

- Who Is on a Multi-Disciplinary Weight-Loss/Obesity Treatment Team and What Are Their Roles?

Introduction

For most people, body image, weight, and self-esteem are personal. We usually don't like to discuss either our weight or our eating habits if we feel that this information will be received in a negative manner. Most people realize when they are gaining weight, but they might not realize just how much weight they have put on. It can be very disheartening for a person to realize that they have gone from "my pants are a little snug," or "maybe they shrunk in the dryer?" to being classified as "obese" or in a "high-risk" category. It is sobering to see "obese" or "severe obesity" listed as a problem in your medical chart. Obesity is a complex, chronic, progressive, and life-threatening disease, especially when left unmanaged; it is not simply an indication that a person lacks discipline or motivation (Blackburn et al, 2008).

Don't despair! The fact that you are even reading this book is a good sign! Accepting that you have obesity is the first—and maybe the most important—step to successful management of your weight. Many dedicated professionals in the medical community are available to help you take steps to lose weight and to achieve a healthy *body mass index* (BMI). This chapter discusses which professionals are best suited to help you face obesity.

Is Multi-Disciplinary Care Right for Me?

Multi-disciplinary care is beneficial for anyone who has found it difficult to lose weight, especially after having already attempted multiple serious efforts to lose weight. People who have just a few pounds to lose and who have not struggled with obesity might have success with lifestyle changes and routine monitoring from a health professional. If you are someone who has been trying to manage your weight through diet and exercise for as long as you can remember (and unable to lose weight), it might be time to consider a more holistic approach that involves medical professionals who are dedicated to your success. Multi-disciplinary care should include making small realistic steps toward establishing a permanent lifestyle change. A loss of only 10% of your weight is associated with significant health benefits. Small changes, such as improving the quality of your diet, adding regular physical activity, and enhancing the quality and duration of your sleep, can add up (Figure 14-1).

The BMI chart is used to determine your level of *risk* in relation to your weight and can help determine what interventions will be best for you now. To calculate your BMI, refer to Chapter 5. Also, many BMI calculators are available on-line (for free).

Classification of Overweight and Obesity by BMI, Waist Circumference, and Associated Disease Risks

	BMI (kg/m^2)	Obesity Class	Disease Risk* Relative to Normal Weight and Waist Circumference Men 102 cm (40 in) or less Women 88 cm (35 in) or less	Men > 102 cm (40 in) Women > 88 cm (35 in)
Underweight	< 18.5			
Normal	18.5–24.9			
Overweight	25.0–29.9		Increased	High
Obesity	30.0–34.9	I	High	Very High
	35.0–39.9	II	Very High	Very High
Extreme Obesity	40.0 +	III	Extremely High	Extremely High

* Disease risk for type 2 diabetes, hypertension, and CVD.
+ Increased waist circumference also can be a marker for increased risk, even in persons of normal weight.

Figure 14-1: Classification of overweight and obesity by BMI, waist circumference, and associated disease risks (from National Institutes of Health "Aim for a Healthy Weight" [https://www.nhlbi.nih.gov/health/educational/lose_wt/BMI/bmi_dis.htm]).

Who Is on a Multi-Disciplinary Weight-Loss/Obesity Treatment Team and What Are Their Roles?

Primary-Care Physician/Family Physician

Hopefully you've already established a relationship with a Primary-Care Physician (PCP) with whom you feel comfortable and can trust. It's important for you to be open and honest with your PCP about your struggles with your weight and concerns about your health. It can be helpful to keep a food journal for a few days and to record your diet, exercise, sleep, and other habits. This could help your PCP assess any areas that might need adjustments. Your PCP will also perform routine screening and discuss your risk factors.

As part of routine screening, your PCP might obtain some lab tests. These lab tests can help to determine the impact of your weight on your health. Your doctor has the final say on what tests will be needed based on your personal health history. Lab tests could include *serum electrolytes, cholesterol levels*, a *lipid profile*, an *electrocardiogram* (EKG) (to look at your heart rhythm), a *hemoglobin A1C* (to get an average of your blood sugar over the past 3 months), *thyroid function tests* (to rule-out hormonal causes of your weight gain), and *liver function tests*.

Endocrinologist

An *endocrinologist* is a doctor who specializes in the hormones of the body and their effects on health. Several hormone problems (e.g., *polycystic ovarian syndrome* [PCOS], *hypothyroidism*) can make it increasingly difficult to lose weight. Endocrinologists can screen for disorders of the thyroid, ovaries, adrenal gland, and pituitary gland disorders to be sure that these are not the cause of your obesity. There are also doctors called *reproductive endocrinologists* who can be helpful for women who find themselves struggling with infertility. Often, weight loss improves fertility, especially in patients with moderate to severe obesity. Reproductive endocrinologists can help with that condition.

Bariatric Surgeon

Bariatric surgeons are physicians who specialize in weight-loss surgery. Bariatric surgery can improve several conditions caused by, or worsened by, obesity. In general, to qualify for bariatric surgery, your BMI must be greater than 40 (or be at least 100 pounds overweight); your BMI is 35 or more and you have at least one obesity-related co-morbidity; or you have been unable to achieve a healthy weight with previous attempts at weight loss. Psychological assessments are often completed before undergoing bariatric surgery. (https://asmbs.org/patients/who-is-a-candidate-for-bariatric-surgery-2017).

When behavioral and lifestyle changes have been unsuccessful for children and adolescents with obesity, more aggressive treatments like medications and possibly bariatric surgery might be required. The most common operations performed in children or adolescents affected by extreme obesity are *Roux-en-Y gastric bypass*, *laparoscopic adjustable gastric banding*, and *vertical sleeve gastrectomy*. Of these procedures, the vertical sleeve gastrectomy is now the most commonly performed weight-loss procedure in the United States. The health-care team evaluates each individual with obesity and carefully weighs the pros and cons of surgery. Some insurance companies will not cover bariatric surgery for children under the age of 18 (https://asmbs.org/patients/adolescent-obesity-2017).

Obesity Medicine Specialist

An *obesity medicine specialist* is a physician who is dedicated to the comprehensive care of people with obesity. They are comfortable using medications, behavioral interventions, and exercise regimens to combat obesity. Obesity medicine specialists receive additional training and certifications to better understand and address the issues that flow from obesity. Obesity medicine specialists understand and agree that obesity is a chronic disease that changes the way your body functions and must be managed over the long term.

Psychiatrist

A psychiatrist is a physician who specializes in the diagnosis and treatment of mental illness, eating disorders, and substance use disorders. Psychiatrists are trained to assess the mental and physical aspects of health problems. Psychiatrists can conduct talk therapy (*psychotherapy*), institute psychosocial interventions, and/or prescribe medications. Psychotherapy can be used to eliminate or control troubling symptoms so that you are better able to focus on addressing your obesity. Obesity can also be caused by medications called *psychotropics* that are used to treat mental disorders. Thus, it is important to include a psychiatrist in your multi-disciplinary obesity team (Chwastiak & Tek, 2014). If you have a psychiatric condition (like depression, anxiety, or bipolar disorder), you might need to continue receiving treatment for those conditions while addressing your obesity and overall physical health.

Psychologist

Psychologists are mental-health professionals who have doctoral-level degrees (PhD, PsyD, or EdD) and are trained to address a person's stress or difficulty in life. As a part of any multi-disciplinary weight-loss program, it can be helpful to understand the underlying causes or behaviors that sabotage success. Before being approved for bariatric surgery, most patients must be evaluated by a mental-health provider. It is vital to understand whether psychological reasons contribute to your weight gain and to problem-solve to prevent them from becoming barriers to success. For instance, binge eating could complicate bariatric surgery; therefore, it is important to address this before undergoing surgery. When problems are unknown or unaddressed, patients might have poor surgical outcomes and fail to achieve their weight-loss goal over the long term.

Registered Dietitian

Dietitians can help develop eating plans that address specific diet quality considerations and can also address nutritional deficiencies that you might have. It is important to have a dietitian who is experienced with treating obesity. Dietitians who have been trained to work with someone who is undergoing bariatric surgery can be particularly useful to address specific nutritional deficiencies. Dietitians can help make sure that you're able to follow dietary guidelines, eat proper portions, and make behavioral changes necessary to address your weight.

Physical Therapist

A *physical therapist* can teach you how to perform exercises that will help you to begin to become more active while losing weight. They are especially useful if you've had trouble with inactivity, or prior injuries, or if you lack knowledge on how to exercise safely. Physical exercise helps maintain weight loss, reduce your stress level, and improve your mood. A physical therapist can help you take the necessary steps to reach your goals while becoming physically stronger. You might discover a world of physical activity (e.g., biking, walking your dog, swimming) that you were previously unable to perform.

Pain Specialist

Unfortunately, chronic pain is associated with obesity for a variety of reasons. A pain specialist can help you with underlying issues that hinder your ability to exercise or function. Depending on your level of chronic pain, it might be difficult to get through the day. Exercise can help you to maintain weight loss and improve your sense of well-being. Pain specialists can help provide you with solutions for difficult-to-control pain while allowing you to focus on your weight loss (Schnitzer, 2017).

Case Manager/Social Worker

When handling difficult situations, related to medical illness or other problems, it can feel as though it is too difficult to manage on your own. You might not know how or where to find the appropriate care. *Case managers* and *social workers* can help you to achieve a better quality of life. There are several types of case managers, including juvenile case managers, mental-health case managers, and social-work case managers, just to name a few. The common ground for most case managers is that they advocate, educate, and provide emotional support for people in need. Case managers can assess your strengths and identify barriers that interfere with success. Case managers are vital to a well-run multi-disciplinary team because they can identify specific areas of need where you require more individualized help from others on the medical team. Case managers can help you understand insurance issues, make timely follow-up appointments, or find resources in the community. (http://www.psychologyschoolguide.net/social-work-careers/case-manager/). Case managers usually determine the best services available and then social workers perform the daily tasks to make sure that your goals will be met. Social workers work closely with you to help provide more regular support and counseling to help you stay on track. They also help make sure that you have access to resources in your community (http://www.casemanagementbasics.com/).

Thus, there are a host of dedicated members of the medical team who can help you address your obesity and struggles. You can begin by speaking with your PCP and determining your specific needs and risk factors. If you are ready to move forward on your weight-loss journey, consider researching the resources provided in this chapter and contacting a weight-management center in your area.

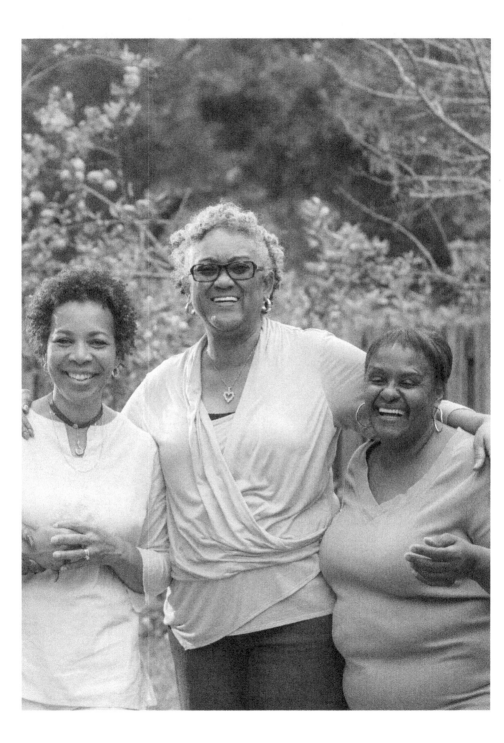

WHAT TYPES OF INTERVENTIONS MIGHT HELP ME AS I ATTEMPT TO LOSE WEIGHT?

Humsini Viswanath, BA, MPH; Elizabeth Hartwig, BA; and
Michelle A. Patriquin, PhD

CHAPTER

In This Chapter

- Why Might I Need Psychological or Social Support While Losing Weight?

- Why Is Psychological Support Important?

- Why Is Social Support Important?

- What Are Group Therapy and Overeaters Anonymous?

- What Is Individual Psychotherapy?

- What Types of Behavioral Interventions Might I Try?

- How Can I Get a Referral for Help in My Community?

Introduction

Eating a healthy diet and exercising sound like easy ways to lose weight, right? Although it sounds simple, losing weight is difficult for many people. This chapter discusses why losing weight can create a mental challenge. It also reviews the various resources that are available to help and support you and how you can obtain that help.

Why Might I Need Psychological or Social Support While Losing Weight?

The relationship between weight gain and mental health is complicated. How do we know which one comes first—the mental-health issues or the weight gain? However, just because you are gaining weight, it doesn't mean that you have mental-health issues or a psychiatric disorder. And, even if you suffer from a mental-health problem, it doesn't mean that you will gain weight. Psychological support and social support while losing weight is important to jumpstart and to maintain your weight-loss efforts.

Why Is Psychological Support Important?

Studies have shown that being diagnosed with overweight, obesity, or severe obesity might be associated with psychiatric conditions (e.g., *major depressive disorder* [MDD], *dysthymia, bipolar disorder*) or personality disorders (e.g., antisocial, avoidant, schizoid, paranoid, obsessive-compulsive personality disorders) (Petry et al, 2008).

Most people with overweight or obesity do not have a mood disorder (e.g., depression). It has been shown, however, that those who seek help for their mood disorder might have excess weight. Additionally, mood disorders are common in those who are seeking help for obesity. Some researchers have suggested that depression might subside after you complete a weight-loss program (e.g., if your depression began after your weight gain), but if you are obese and suffer from a mood disorder, both need to be treated for effective weight loss (McElroy et al, 2004).

Severe obesity is not only associated with depression, but also anxiety disorders, particularly in women (Scott et al, 2008). With anxiety comes an increased level of *cortisol*, a hormone that increases your appetite (especially for sweet food) and stimulates growth of fat deposits in your abdominal area (see Figure 15-1). Increased levels of cortisol have been found in individuals who are obese or have a large waist circumference (Jackson et al, 2017).

Difficulties with emotional regulation are also associated with higher weight (Kass et al, 2017). Although you might not be aware of it, one of your main coping skills when you are stressed or depressed could be *emotional eating*. Emotional eating involves eating without being hungry. You might eat for comfort when you are stressed, sad, or angry. It is important to learn effective coping skills to deal with stress and depression instead of emotional eating. Rather than eating to cope, healthy coping skills include deep breathing, the practice of *yoga*, or use of other relaxation techniques.

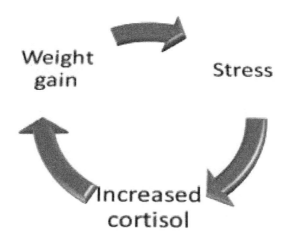

Figure 15-1: Cortisol, weight gain, and the stress cycle.

Children, especially girls with overweight and obesity, have lower self-esteem. Children with low self-esteem usually feel lonely, sad, and engage in risky behaviors (e.g., smoking cigarettes, drinking alcohol) (Strauss, 2000). Additionally, low self-esteem is linked to poor *body image*. As such, the best way to assist with weight loss in adolescents is to promote proper eating habits and physical activity, while focusing on positive attributes through psychological support (Peas et al, 2000). Whether you have a psychiatric disorder or not, psychological support during attempts to lose weight is beneficial for maintaining a healthy outlook on the weight-loss process.

Why Is Social Support Important?

Most activities are more fun when done with someone else. Individuals who commit to weight-loss programs with a friend obtain benefits, as well. Working out with a friend can increase your commitment and your enjoyment from the program. Roughly two-thirds of those who joined a weight-loss program with a friend maintained their weight 6 months after the program ended, as compared to those who joined the program alone (Wing & Jeffery, 1999). For children, it helps to have peers and family members working toward the same goal, all committed to the program. Increased family satisfaction and how happy a parent is with their life is associated with a child's successful weight loss (White et al, 2004). Whether you are trying to lose weight or you know someone who is losing weight, it is beneficial to have a support system to facilitate motivation and to stay positive during and after the process.

What Are Group Therapy and Overeaters Anonymous?

Several types of therapy are beneficial for weight loss. You can participate in group therapy or individual therapy depending on your preference. You can even combine them. Within group therapy and individual therapy, there are a variety of approaches.

Group Therapy

Group therapy usually involves five or more individuals with one or more psychologists or other licensed mental-health professionals (e.g., licensed clinical social worker, psychiatrist). The groups typically meet at least once a week for an hour or more to discuss a specific topic, emotional response, or behavior. According to the *American Psychological Association* (APA), group therapy is beneficial for several reasons:

- Members of the group form a support network and are there to help you with ideas on how to deal with certain situations.

- You gain perspective on your problems by listening to the struggles of others.

- You learn from different people who come from diverse backgrounds and have varied personalities. Group therapy helps you put yourself in someone else's shoes and think about different approaches when you're facing a problem.

If you are interested in group therapy, one popular type of group therapy is *Overeaters Anonymous* (OA). It is a nonprofit organization (supported solely by donations) that is led by volunteers. OA believes that obesity results from compulsive eating linked with negative emotions. OA's premise is that excess food consumption has led to excess weight, and this book has taught you that obesity is much more complex than evaluating excess food consumption. OA takes an emotional and spiritual approach using the *12-step program*.

However, OA states that atheists and agnostics are welcome. Each OA group is different, so it is important to meet with several of them to see which one fits you best. OA also utilizes the following tools for recovery:

- A plan for eating: for example, abstain from compulsive eating

- A sponsor, who guides you and encourages you to call when you suspect you will relapse

- Regular meetings that help you identify your problems

- Writing about how you are feeling

- Reading literature that reinforces the 12-step program and *12 traditions*

- An action plan with attainable goals

- Anonymity so that you do not feel vulnerable

- Service: if you help others within the group, it will help your recovery

Unfortunately, no studies have shown the effectiveness of OA; however, that doesn't mean it isn't an effective option for helping you to lose weight. It will be very helpful if you feel like you need emotional support when you are trying to lose weight (Tsai & Wadden, 2005).

Other Group Therapy Options

There are a variety of ways to participate in group therapy sessions. You can join non-medical commercial programs, organized self-help programs, internet-based commercial programs, or medically supervised proprietary programs. Most weight-loss programs have not been studied extensively, except for non-medical commercial groups (e.g., Weight Watchers), where individuals were shown to lose weight; however, there was a lot of attrition from the program. Table 15-1 provides you with information about each weight-loss program that includes group therapy (Tsai & Wadden, 2005).

Table 15-1: Weight Loss Programs that Include Group Therapy

Program	Type	Staff Qualifications	Diet	Physical Activity	Behavior Modification	Support
Weight Watchers	Non-medical commercial	Successful program completer	Low-calorie; prepare own meals	"Get Moving" booklet	Behavioral weight-control methods	Weekly group sessions
Health Management Resources	Medically supervised	Physician or health-care provider	Very low-calorie; uses meal replacement products	Walking and calorie counting charts	In lifestyle classes; skills and accountability stressed	Group sessions, weekly classes, telephone support
OPTIFAST	Medically supervised	Physician or health-care provider	Low-calorie; uses meal replacement products	Taught in lifestyle classes	In lifestyle classes; stress and social support emphasized	Group sessions, weekly classes, telephone support
eDiets.com	Internet-based commercial	Company-trained counselor or dieticians	Low-calorie via "virtual dietitian"; prepare own meals	Seminar included	eDiets.com University; stress management focus	Individual and group internet support
Take Off Pounds Sensibly	Organized self-help	Group leader elected by local chapter	Low-calorie; exchange recipes	Make plans with health-care provider	In curriculum	Weekly group sessions
Overeaters Anonymous	Organized self-help	Volunteer chapter leaders	No specific recommendations	Make plans with health-care provider	12-step program	Weekly group sessions and there are sponsors

What Is Individual Psychotherapy?

Individual therapy, or one-on-one therapy, occurs when an individual and his or her psychologist or other licensed mental-health professional work together. Even when one-on-one psychotherapy is embarked upon, several different types of therapy can be employed; the strategy depends on the training and theoretical orientation of the psychologist or licensed mental-health professional and what will work for the individual (APA). Types of therapy includes:

Cognitive-behavioral therapy (CBT)
> This is a practical approach in which you track your behaviors and reactions to certain events and use new skills that your therapist teaches you.

Psychoanalytic therapy and a humanistic approach
> You will spend time talking to the psychologist or other licensed mental-health professional to get to the root cause of your problem.

Even though individual therapy might be less daunting than group therapy in the beginning, it has been shown that group therapy can reduce weight and body mass more than individual therapy (Renjilian et al, 2001).

What Types of Behavioral Interventions Might I Try?

Behavioral interventions lead to better outcomes than educational interventions alone (e.g., reading pamphlets or websites on nutrition and physical activity). This is because educational interventions tend to teach people what to change and not *how* to change. Behavioral interventions often focus on problem-solving tools (Figure 15-2) to help people understand what leads them toward unwanted behaviors (like over-eating) and show them how interventions can change behaviors. An example of this is shown in Figure 15-3 (Foster et al, 2005).

Goal Setting

• Set specific goals, that are not overly ambitious.

Self-monitoring

• Ask yourself what your barriers and challenges are for changing your behavior.

Feedback and reinforcement

• Get feedback from your mental health provider to figure out what you need to change and achieve your goal.

Positive "self-talk"

• Improve your optimism and self-esteem by setting realistic goals and achieving them (e.g., eating fruit instead of cake) or get help from others (e.g., group therapy, family members, or friends).

Incentives

• Use incentives to help change behavior (e.g., workplace incentives to help employees regain and maintain their physical health).

Figure 15-2: An example of the steps involved in CBT.

Among behavioral interventions for weight loss, combined behavioral interventions, exercise, and diet is better than any one approach alone (Johns et al, 2014); for example, CBT along with exercise and diet produce better results than just using exercise (Shaw et al, 2005). Most behavioral interventions incorporate CBT-based steps. To get a sense of how CBT works, look at the different steps shown in Figure 15-3 (Strecher et al, 1995).

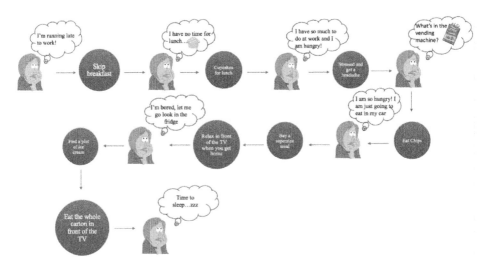

Figure 15-3: Cartoon depicting a behavioral intervention.

Although CBT focuses on goal-setting and behavioral changes, it does not necessarily address psychological conditions (e.g., depression, anxiety) or issues that underlie obesity (e.g., stigma, isolation, low self-esteem) (Shaw et al, 2005) mindfulness-based interventions (Figure 15-4), can help to improve eating behaviors (binge eating or emotional eating), depression, eating attitudes, anxiety, and BMI (Rogers et al, 2017).

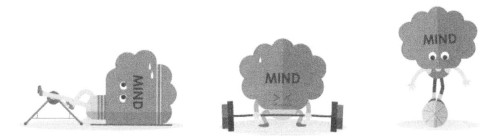

Figure 15-4: Schematic of mindfulness-based therapies.

Mindfulness is the awareness that comes from paying attention to internal and external sensations and thoughts, in the present, and non-judgmentally seeing things as they are (Teasdale & Segal, 2007). Most mindfulness therapies include the following:

- Classroom activities: for example, lectures, discussions, and exercises

- Lessons on meditation

- The opportunity to practice (for at least 30 minutes) by yourself

Through these different components, you learn how to accept your circumstances and emotions, even if they are very challenging. You can become more aware of your emotions and be less reactive to situations; this will allow you to make better choices that align with your health goals. You will also learn how to practice mindful eating (involving eating slowly, being aware of your hunger, learning how to savor your food, and knowing when you're satiated) while also practicing self-acceptance (Kristeller & Wolever, 2010). Through becoming more aware of your emotions and practicing mindful eating, you will learn how to deal with your emotions and to create healthier habits to deal with your emotions, rather than suppressing emotions with food.

It is important to remember that mindfulness strategies are helpful, but they are more effective when combined with an appropriate diet and exercise regimen along with behavioral components of CBT (Olson & Emery, 2015).

How Can I Get a Referral for Help in My Community?

There are several paths that you can take to help with your weight-loss goals. Determining the best therapy option for your weight-loss plan can seem daunting; however, health professionals can guide you through the process. You can find more information about weight-management groups from your local hospital or you can talk with your primary-care physician to obtain a referral to the type of support group or individual therapy that is most appropriate for you. If you are interested in individual therapy, you can do the following:

- Ask your physician or another health professional for a referral

- Call or search on-line (through your local or state psychological association) to find a licensed psychologist or other licensed mental-health professional

- Use the APA's professional locator at http://locator.apa.org.

- Use the *Association of Behavioral and Cognitive Therapies* (ABCT) therapist locator at http://www.findcbt.org/xFAT/.

If you are interested in group therapy, you can do the following:

- Contact non-medical commercial groups (e.g., Weight Watchers, Jenny Craig), internet-based commercial programs (e.g., eDiets.com), organized self-help groups (e.g., Overeaters Anonymous); for these programs you do not need a referral. You can go on-line and find a location for the in-person groups and get started. It might be beneficial to try out different groups to see which one is the best fit for you.

- Contact medical weight-loss programs. Because these cater to severe cases (typically involving obesity-related health complications), most of them require a physician referral because patients go on very low-calorie diets, for which medical supervision is required.

In sum, psychological and social support are key components to help you reach your weight-loss goals. Group therapy, individual therapy, or a combination of the two, can provide meaningful support. CBT can teach you *how* you will implement your weight-loss plan. Further, mindfulness-based interventions address psychological issues that underlie weight gain and provide access to other resources. These psychological interventions can provide the support needed to ensure that your chances of reaching your weight-loss goals are maximized.

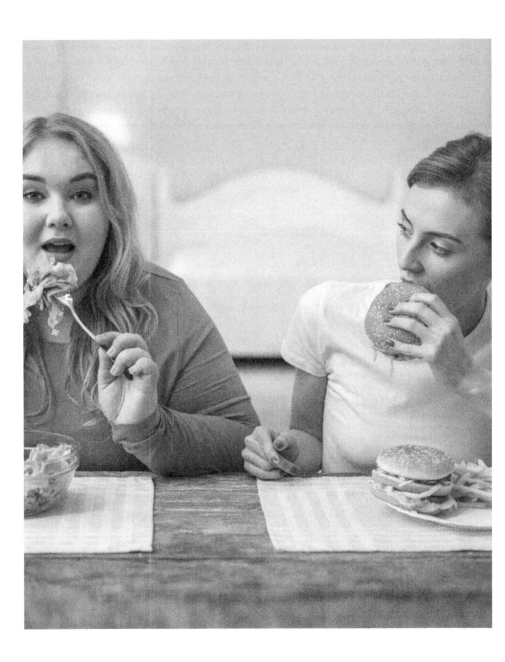

WEIGHT BIAS AND STIGMA

Fatima Cody Stanford, MD, MPH, MPA, FAAP, FTOS

CHAPTER

In This Chapter

- Have You Been the Perpetrator or the Recipient of Weight Bias?

- Is There a Relationship Between Weight Bias and Poor Education About Obesity?

- What Are the Common Forms of Bias in the United States?

- How Early in Life Does Weight Bias Develop (and Why)?

- How Does Paternal Influence Affect Weight Bias in Children?

- Is There a Relationship Among Weight Bias, Teasing, and Psychosocial Functioning?

- What Is the Relationship Among Weight Bias Internalization, Metabolic Syndrome, and Mental Health?

- How Do Weight Stigma, Internalization, and Coping Strategies Relate to One Another?

- Do Health Professionals Experience, Convey, or Manifest Weight Bias?

- What Is the Relationship Between Weight Stigma and Health Outcomes?

- How Can Exercise Be Promoted Without Promoting Weight Bias?

continued

- Is There a Relationship Among Weight Bias, Educational Opportunities, and Employability?

- What Is the Impact of Reality TV Shows and Weight Bias?

- Is There a Relationship Between Weight Bias and Stigma in the United States and Abroad?

- Are there Laws Against Obesity Discrimination?

Introduction

As obesity rates continue to rise in the United States and throughout the world, the bias toward those individuals who struggle with weight also climbs. *Weight bias*, the discrimination against those who carry excess weight, can be both explicit or implicit. *Explicit weight bias* is bias toward a person who carries excess weight, and the holder of the bias is aware of the discrimination that they wield against the overweight person. With *implicit bias*, the individual who harbors the bias is often unaware that they have bias against persons with overweight or obesity. Unfortunately, the bias against those with overweight and obesity is widely accepted and has become one of the most prevalent forms of bias. So why is weight bias important? Why have we chosen to dedicate an entire chapter in this text to weight bias? It is time to find out.

In this chapter, we do the following:

- Explore how weight bias and stigma contribute to energy storage

- Learn how early life interactions influence weight bias

- Determine the negative impact of weight bias on health outcomes

- Acknowledge how health professionals (much like those in the public) harbor implicit and explicit weight bias

- Look at national and international trends in weight bias and its affect on quality of life on the individuals who experience such bias.

To help focus your learning on weight bias, we pose three multiple-choice questions at the beginning of this chapter regarding the topic of weight bias. By the end of this chapter you should be able to answer them correctly.

Question 1. What is the average age at which infants/toddlers begin to demonstrate signs of weight bias?

a.   12 months

b.   20 months

c.   32 months

d.   48 months

Question 2. Weight stigma has not been associated with which of the following in individuals?

a.   Disordered eating

b.   *Metabolic syndrome* (a predisposition to type 2 diabetes mellitus)

c.   *Hypertension* (elevated blood pressure)

d.   High triglyceride levels (elevated levels of bad cholesterol)

e.   Low levels of *high-density lipoproteins* (HDL; a type of good cholesterol)

Question 3. Which country has the highest level of weight bias?

a.   Australia

b.   Canada

c.   Iceland

d.   United States

e.   All countries have similar levels of weight bias

Have You Been the Perpetrator or the Recipient of Weight Bias?

Let's take a moment to look back at your life. In your lifetime, have you ever discriminated against an individual because they had overweight or obesity? If you didn't explicitly discriminate, did you pass judgement about an individual and their weight status? Or, maybe you are an individual who was the recipient of such bias? Have you been made to feel unwelcome due to your weight? How did that make you feel? After reading the aforementioned questions, it is likely that you have either been the perpetrator or the recipient of weight bias. We should make strides to reduce weight bias because it leads to a worse quality of life for the recipients of such bias. I am frequently asked, "Doc, but isn't it often just fun and games? I really don't mean any harm by making fun of people who are just 'fat.'" Well, it might not seem harmful to you, but for the person who experiences such bias it can have a life-long impact.

Is There a Relationship Between Weight Bias and Poor Education About Obesity?

One of the primary reasons that weight bias and stigma continue to be so pervasive in our society is because of inadequate knowledge about obesity. Despite the belief that weight regulation is all about "calories in and calories out," we know that weight regulation is much more complex; this explains why some people gain and retain weight quite easily, whereas others have difficulty in gaining weight. There are a variety of contributing factors to obesity that are both internal and external to an individual (see Figure 16-1).

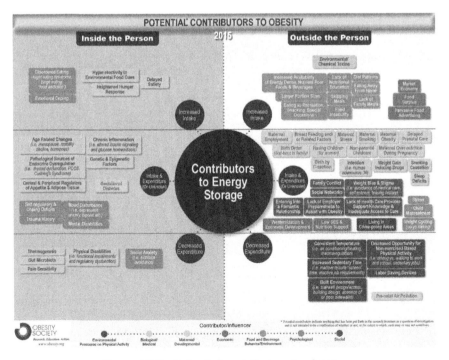

Figure 16-1: Potential contributors to obesity.

As noted in Table 16-1, contributors to obesity can be characterized in several ways; these conditions affect how a much a person eats and how many calories they can burn.

Table 16-1: Contributors to Obesity

Biological/Medical Factors
    Age-related changes (e.g., menopause)
    Genetics
    Medications that cause weight gain

Food and Beverage Behavior/Environmental Factors
    Diet patterns
    Skipping meals
    Large-portion sizes

Maternal/Developmental Factors
    Maternal/paternal obesity
    Maternal stress
    Delayed pre-natal care

Social Factors
    Weight bias and stigma
    Family conflict
    Social networks

Psychological Factors
    Mood and anxiety disorders (e.g., depression, anxiety, bipolar disorder)
    Trauma history
    Stress

Economic Factors
    Low socioeconomic status (SES) and support
    Pervasive food advertising
    Westernization and economic development

Environmental Pressures on Physical Activity
    Built environment
    Increased sedentary time
    Decreased opportunities for non-exercise-related physical activity (e.g., walking to work *versus* driving to work)

What Are the Common Forms of Bias in the United States?

The two most common forms of bias in the United States are race bias and weight bias. An article in the *Washington Post* noted that searches for "three black teenagers" on the most popular search engine, Google, were met with stereotyped pictures of black teenage males—mugshots (Guarino, 2016). When a similar search was conducted with the search terms of "three white teenagers," the search returned pictures of smiling white teenagers. Similarly, in a *Glamour* magazine article, readers were shown pictures of two blond White women; one had a thin body type and the other had a heavy body type (Driesbach, 2012). The adjectives used to describe the thin woman were superficial, ambitious, confident, vain, conceited, and mean, whereas the adjectives used to describe the woman with the heavier body type were lazy, insecure, undisciplined, passive, and careless.

In a study that evaluated the differences among Black, Hispanic, and White women in the United States to ascertain the likelihood of explicit and implicit weight bias, Black women had less explicit weight bias than did White women (Hubner et al, 2016). Despite having lower levels of explicit weight bias, they had high levels of implicit weight bias that was strongly associated with their ethnic identity. Black women with a lower ethnic identity were more likely to have negative implicit bias than were those who had a stronger ethnic identity. These are examples of how bias appears in our society.

How Early in Life Does Weight Bias Develop (and Why)?

A recent study sought to determine how early in life children begin to demonstrate weight bias and how this is influenced by their mother's own bias against individuals with excess weight. In this study, 70 mother–infant pairs were examined to determine their preference for a normal or heavy body type by allowing the infants and toddlers to view, in random order, pairs of individuals with normal weight status or overweight or obesity in which their viewing time (preferential viewing time) was measured (Spiel et al, 2016). Older infants (average age, approximately 11 months) displayed a preference for individuals with obesity, whereas older toddlers (average age, 32 months) displayed a preference for individuals with normal weight status. The bias against individuals with overweight and obesity was strongly related to their mother's weight bias, such that the infants and toddlers with mothers with a strong bias against people with overweight and obesity had a much higher likelihood of having a similar bias.

How Does Paternal Influence Affect Weight Bias in Children?

Weight bias in mothers strongly influences weight bias in toddlers. However, do we know how parental weight bias influences preschool-aged children? One study evaluated more than 270 children (3-year-olds) and their parents to determine whether the parents' beliefs about body size and dieting influenced their children over the course of 1 year (Tanneberger & Ciupitu-Plath, 2016); the children had more negative associations about larger body types. Fathers had a strong influence on their boys and their weight bias, whereas there was not a strong association with either parents' beliefs and their daughter's likelihood of having weight bias.

Is There a Relationship Among Weight Bias, Teasing, and Psychosocial Functioning?

A study of 1,047 boys between the ages of 7 and 11 in Germany sought to determine how a boy's weight status (as defined by their *body mass index* [BMI]) at the start of the study influenced weight bias and teasing later in life (Alberga et al, 2017). They found that boys who had weighed more were more likely to have experienced weight teasing, weight-bias internalization, and restrained their eating. If a boy was teased about his weight, he was more likely to have emotional and conduct problems. For those boys who internalized the weight bias they experienced, they were more likely to have emotional problems and restrained eating. This study demonstrated that a boy's weight status and the bias that they were subjected to affected their psychosocial heath.

What Is the Relationship Among Weight Bias Internalization, Metabolic Syndrome, and Mental Health?

A recent study sought to determine whether weight bias internalization was associated with the likelihood of having metabolic syndrome (a predisposition to developing type 2 diabetes mellitus) (Rudolph and Hilbert, 2017). In this study of 178 obese adults in a weight-loss trial, investigators measured blood pressure, waist circumference, *fasting blood sugar* levels (glucose), *triglyceride* levels (one of the bad cholesterols), and *high-density lipoprotein* (HDL) cholesterol levels (the good cholesterol). The study concluded that people who had higher levels of weight bias internalization had a greater likelihood of developing metabolic syndrome and high triglyceride levels. Additionally, persons who experienced weight bias developed stress that was a contributor to weight gain as well as disordered and maladaptive behaviors.

How Do Weight Stigma, Internalization, and Coping Strategies Relate to One Another?

In this chapter, we have already learned that weight bias and stigma is associated with obesity and its co-morbidities as well as negative health outcomes that further worsen the weight and health of individuals who have excess weight. It must also be noted that women and minority populations have higher rates of obesity in the United States. Despite the higher rates of obesity in these communities, little research has been done to explore obesity's relationship to weight bias and stigma. In a study of 2,378 individuals, women were more likely to have weight bias internalization as men (Himmelstein et al, 2017). Black men and women were less likely to internalize weight bias than were White men and women.

Black women were least likely (when compared to White women and Hispanic women) to cope with weight stigma with disordered eating, in contrast to Hispanic women, who were most likely to demonstrate signs of disordered eating when they internalized weight bias. Surprisingly, Black men were more likely to cope with weight stigma with eating. This study demonstrated that weight bias and stigma are present in racial groups, and racial and gender groups differ regarding how they cope with weight stigma.

Do Health Professionals Experience, Convey, or Manifest Weight Bias?

Perhaps one might think that medical students would have a low likelihood of demonstrating weight bias compared to those in the general population; however, this is far from true. A study conducted at Wake Forest Medical School tested third-year medical students with the Weight Implicit Association Test (IAT) and found that more than one-third of the students demonstrated a strong bias toward persons who carried excess weight, and that more than two-thirds of the students were unaware of their biases (demonstrating a high level of implicit bias) (Pantenburg et al, 2013). A more extensive study evaluated 1,795 medical students from 49 medical schools in the United States to determine how weight bias evolved between their first and fourth years of medical school (Puhl et al, 2015). They also compared the outcomes to those of nearly 400,000 (397,600) persons in the general public who visited www.projectimplicit.org between 2010 and 2013. The investigators measured implicit weight bias with the IAT. Although implicit weight bias decreased dramatically during medical school training, investigators found that explicit weight bias increased and paralleled the increase in explicit weight bias in the public. The authors of the study concluded that medical schools might reduce students' weight biases by doing the following:

- Increasing positive contact between students and patients with obesity

- Eliminating unprofessional role-modeling by faculty members and residents

- Altering curricula that focused on treating difficult patients.

In an in-depth evaluation of implicit weight bias in medical students, using Implicit Relational Assessment Procedure (IRAP) assessments, comparisons were made between first- and third-year medical students. Of the 325 assessments, 40 were completed by the same group of medical students in their first and third years of medical school. There was little change in implicit attitudes toward individuals classified as overweight, but there was a significant improvement in implicit bias toward persons with obesity. In the group of 40 students who were followed from their first to third years of medical school, there was a substantial improvement in bias toward persons classified as overweight, but there was not a significant improvement in weight bias with respect to bias toward patients with obesity.

In a recent review of the medical literature to determine whether there were any consistently used strategies to reduce weight bias in health professionals (Baker et al, 2016), researchers found that bias was reduced in weight professionals with enhanced knowledge of the causes of obesity; however, there was no evidence to support long-term benefits of having this knowledge.

When individuals are obese they often recognize that health providers have a bias against them, and they receive threatening environmental cues within the health-care setting; these align with health-care provider's bias (Phelan et al, 2015). As a result of such weight bias, patients will avoid care, mistrust health providers, demonstrate poor adherence with recommendations, become stressed, and have poor patient–provider interactions.

In concert with the health provider's stereotypes of the patient and biased decision making, these attitudes lead to negative patient outcomes.

What Is the Relationship Between Weight Stigma and Health Outcomes?

Weight stigma leads to stress, and stress affects eating and physical activity (e.g., binge eating, increased caloric consumption, maladaptive weight control, disordered eating, motivation for physical activity, and physical activity) and physiologic reactivity (e.g., increased levels of *C-reactive protein* [an inflammatory marker in the blood], *cortisol* [a stress hormone], *A1C levels* [*hemoglobin A1C* which conveys the average blood sugar over the prior 3-month period], elevated blood pressure) (Allison et al, 2016). Weight stigma also affects the delivery of health services (e.g., poor patient adherence, less trust of health providers, avoidance of follow-up care, delay in preventive health screenings, poor communication). The negative impact on eating and health behaviors, physiologic reactivity, and health-care services leads to further weight gain that causes impaired psychological health and distress (e.g., depression, anxiety, low self-esteem, poor body image, substance abuse, suicidal ideation) as well as physiological health and distress (e.g., poor blood sugar control, less effective chronic disease self-management, more advanced and poorly controlled chronic disease, lower health-related quality of life).

How Can Exercise Be Promoted Without Promoting Weight Bias?

Although health education campaigns aim to prevent and reduce obesity, they often contain weight-stigmatizing visual content that often leads to unintended negative health consequences (Phelan et al, 2015). In a quest to identify non-stigmatizing visual content investigators used an on-line sample of 483 women who viewed several scenarios: a woman with obesity portrayed stereotypically (e.g., eating pizza); a woman with obesity exercising (a counter-stereotypical portrayal); a woman with obesity portrayed neutrally; or a lean woman exercising. Persons with obesity who viewed the portrayal in a neutral way were less likely to elicit expressions of weight bias attitudes and to have higher reports of exercise-liking/comfort. Among persons of normal weight, images portraying women with obesity in a stereotypical or counter-stereotypical fashion increased the likelihood of negative stereotypes as compared to lean images. The study concluded that neutral portrayals of individuals might be an effective route to promote exercise without perpetuating stigma.

Is There a Relationship Among Weight Bias, Educational Opportunities, and Employability?

In a study of students applying for graduate-level psychology programs, a higher BMI significantly predicted fewer post-interview offers of admission into psychology graduate programs; this relationship was stronger for female applicants (Carels et al, 2013). The BMI was not related to the overall quality or the number of stereotypically weight-related adjectives in letters of recommendation, but a higher BMI was related to more positive adjectives in letters.

In a recent study published in *Obesity Surgery*, 154 participants viewed an image of a normal-weight woman and rated their impression of her (Durso et al, 2015). They then rated their impression of her image with excess weight after learning how she had previously gained and subsequently lost weight. Participants rated the individual less favorably (e.g., perceived employability if they thought the individual who once carried excess weight lost weight through surgery *versus* diet and exercise).

What Is the Impact of Reality TV Shows and Weight Bias?

In a study in *Obesity*, 59 participants were assigned to an experimental group (i.e., they viewed one episode of *The Biggest Loser*) or a control group (i.e., they viewed one episode of a nature reality show) (Gujral et al, 2012). The levels of weight bias of the study participants were measured by the IAT, the Obese Person Trait Survey (OPTS), and the Anti-fat Attitudes scale (AFA) at baseline and one week after viewing the episodes. Participants in the experimental group had significantly higher levels of dislike of individuals with overweight and obesity and more strongly believed that weight was within one's control after the experiment.

Is There a Relationship Between Weight Bias and Stigma in the United States and Abroad?

In an assessment of countries and their weight bias and stigma, investigators studied bias in Australia, Canada, Iceland, and the United States (Raves et al, 2005). The extent of weight bias was consistent across all four countries. Attributions of behavioral causes of obesity and beliefs that obesity is attributable to a lack of willpower and personal responsibility lead to stronger bias. The magnitude of weight bias was stronger among men and among individuals without family or friends who had experienced this form of bias.

Are there Laws Against Obesity Discrimination?

Weight discrimination is prevalent, and the need for anti-discrimination legislation rises with more pervasive practices of discrimination. Public support of weight-related anti-discrimination laws or policies in Germany, Iceland, and the United States has been studied (Paxton and Damiano, 2017). Questionnaires were administered to ascertain public support for general and employment-specific weight-related anti-discrimination policies, weight-based victimization, and weight-bias internalization. Although more than half of the German sample agreed with anti-discrimination policies, general anti-discrimination laws received lower support than did employment-specific laws. Support for policies considering obesity as a physical disability was greatest in Germany, whereas support for employment-specific anti-discrimination laws was lower in Germany than in the United States and in Iceland. Total support for weight-related anti-discrimination policies was predicted by lower age, female gender, overweight or obese status, residence in Germany, church membership, and readiness to vote in elections.

Conclusions

- Weight stigma has a negative impact on the health and psychological health of patients who struggle with obesity.

- Weight bias develops in infancy.

- Maternal and paternal anti-fat bias influences children.

- Weight bias can be mitigated by proper training of health professionals.

- Efforts to reduce weight bias can improve the health and quality of life of those who struggle with overweight and obesity.

Answers to the In-Text Questions

1. c.   32 months

2. e.   Low levels of *high-density lipoproteins* (HDL; a type of good cholesterol)

3. e.   All countries have similar levels of weight bias

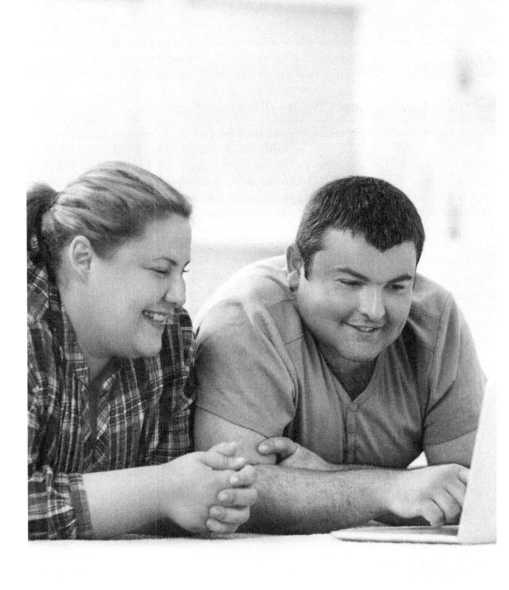

Where Can I Turn For Additional Information On Obesity And Its Treatment?

Slyvia Gonsahn-Bollie, MD

CHAPTER

In This Chapter

- How Can I Become an Obesity Expert?
- Where Can I Go for Reliable Obesity Information?
- Where Can I Find Reliable Information on Weight-Loss Programs, Diets, and Organizations?
- What Internet Sites Can I Use to Learn More About Obesity?

Introduction

There was a time when encyclopedias were the go-to source of reliable information. Though there was a delay in receiving updated information until the next publication of the encyclopedia, you could always trust that the information provided was well researched and reliable. In today's world, we are flooded with information on the internet and via social media. Unfortunately, it is not always reliable, especially with regard to information about weight loss (Modave, 2014). As health-care consumers, it is essential for us to know how to find reliable information, to avoid potentially harmful advice, and to make the smart decisions regarding weight loss and weight management. This chapter helps you to avoid some of the common pitfalls related to inaccurate obesity-related information by addressing the following questions:

- How can I become my own obesity expert?

- Where can I turn for reliable obesity-related information?

- Where can I find reliable information on weight-loss programs, diets, and organizations?

- What internet sites can I use to learn more about obesity?

How Can I Become an Obesity Expert?

When seeking to become an obesity expert, the first question to ask is not "*How?*" but "*Why?*" You should ask yourself: "Why do you want to be an obesity expert?" "Is it for personal or professional use?" After you determine that, you can identify which educational resources you need to develop your expertise about obesity so that you can conquer obesity.

Developing Expertise for Personal Use

If you want to become an obesity expert for personal use, it is important for you to know yourself well. Begin by reflecting on your own weight-management experience. What has been effective (i.e., what has led to weight loss?)? What has not been effective in the short or long term? Evaluate your lifestyle to identify potential barriers to your weight-loss journey. Following self-reflection, you are ready to create your own customized obesity management plan. The next step is to find reliable sources of information to facilitate your plan. We discuss how to find trustworthy sources in the next section.

Developing Professional Expertise

To become a professional obesity expert, begin by evaluating your professional credentials (see Figure 17-1).

- What is your highest level of education?

- Are you willing to pursue additional training in obesity management?

- Do you have any professional experience with obesity management?

Certification Type	High School	Some College/ Associate Degree	College Graduate	Dietician: Registered or Non-Registered	Professional Degree (R.D.,R.N. NP, PA, Master's.)	Doctoral Degree (Ph.D.)	Physician (D.O., M.D.)
Health Coach- International Consortium For Health & Wellness Coaching Website: http://ichwc.org/approved-programs/	✔	✔	✔	✔	✔	✔	✔
Health Coach-American Council on Exercise Website: https://www.acefitness.org/fitness-certifications/health-coach-certification/how-to-become-a-health-coach.aspx		✔	✔	✔	✔	✔	✔
Commission on Dietetic Registration Interdisciplinary Specialist Certification in Obesity and Weight Management Website: https://www.cdrnet.org/interdisciplinary				✔			
American Association of Bariatric Counselors Website: https://aabc-certification.org/how-to-become-certified/				✔	✔	✔	✔
American Board of Obesity Medicine Website: http://www.abom.org/							✔
American Society for Metabolic and Bariatric Surgery Website: https://asmbs.org/professional-education/fellowship					✔ (Certified Bariatric Nurses)		✔
World Obesity Federation SCOPE (Specialist Certification of Obesity Professional Education) Website: https://www.worldobesity.org/scope/certification/			✔	✔	✔	✔	✔

Figure 17-1: Possible routes for obtaining expertise in obesity medicine based on your education level.

It is also important to highlight the following:

- Collaborative certifications are being developed to enhance obesity education.

- There is a paucity of advanced obesity training options for clinicians and researchers.

- A key collaborative certification being developed is the *Certification Board of Obesity Educators*. The goal of this certification is to create a standardized obesity counseling educational platform that can be developed by a broad range of health-care providers as *Certified Obesity Educators*. The target specialties include "physicians, optometrists and podiatrists, registered physician assistants, registered nurses, nurse practitioners, registered dietitians, pharmacists, registered clinical exercise physiologists, physical therapists, occupational therapists, health educators, clinical psychologists, and clinical social workers." (CBOE, 2017)

In the United States, many physicians are underprepared to manage obesity effectively (Talwalker, 2016). Because there is little training available on obesity in medical schools and *residency training programs* (Block, 2003), physicians must seek out additional training on their own. Although, the *American Board of Obesity Medicine* offers a pathway for board certification for qualified physicians, there are very few Obesity Medicine fellowships available. As of 2017, the following Obesity Medicine fellowship programs include (but are not limited to):

- Harvard Medical School Obesity Medicine and Nutrition Fellowship

- Nemours Pediatric Obesity Fellowship

- University of Texas Health Center for Obesity Medicine and Metabolic Performance

- Boston University Medical Center Obesity Medicine Fellowship

- Weill Cornell Medical Center Obesity Medicine Fellowship

- New York University Obesity Medicine Fellowship

For physicians and graduate students who desire research opportunities more options are available. As of 2017, the following obesity research programs exist in the United States:

- University of Alabama-Birmingham

- University of Arizona, Nutritional Sciences Graduate Program, Training Grant in Obesity Research

- Centers for Disease Control & Prevention Nutrition and Obesity Fellowship

- Harvard Training Program in Nutrition and Metabolism

- Johns Hopkins Obesity Research in General Internal Medicine Fellowship

- Minnesota Obesity Prevention Training (MnOPT)

- Yale Program for Obesity, Weight, and Eating Research (POWER)

Where Can I Go for Reliable Obesity Information?

The accuracy of weight-loss information found on an internet search can be as low as 5% (Modave, 2014). Most sources of accurate information on weight loss are found on government sites (e.g., ".gov" or ".org"), medical sites (or obesity medical sources use the resources listed later in this chapter), or university sites (i.e., ".edu").

When reading weight-loss advice, look for the following information:

- Is it consistent with previous weight-loss advice?

- If it is "new," what is the information based on? Specifically, you should look at the scientific study that was done to gather the information.

If you are evaluating the scientific study, use the following as a guide:

What kind of study was it?

Randomized controlled trials (RCTs) are considered the "gold standard" of scientific research (Bothwell, 2016). However, these studies are costly in time and money, so other study types are often conducted and include *observational, case-control,* and *prospective cohort* studies. One major limitation of these studies is that they are often small, so they can generate *false positive* associations that would not be observed in a larger study. One way to correct this is to do a *meta-analysis.* This type of study uses statistical tools to pool the results of smaller studies to derive stronger evidence (Haidich, 2010). Meta-analyses are useful to see whether the health intervention/diet is statistically significant on a larger scale.

Does the study apply to you or to your lifestyle?

For this, you want to read about the study population. First, you need to know whether the study was conducted on humans? You'd be surprised to know that for some breaking news stories, this information was gleaned from animal studies. If humans were the study subjects, look at their characteristics, such as age and sex. This can have significant implications when it comes to applicability to your weight-loss experience. Lastly, look at the intervention used. For instance, if the subjects were exercising for 5 hours each day and eating only 600 kcals per day, this won't be a realistic weight-loss intervention in your daily life.

Were there any conflicts of interest among the authors or investigators?

A conflict of interest occurs when the study's authors have relationships that might bias the results. This is usually in the form of a financial relationship.

When in doubt, talk to your doctor, health-care provider, or a reliable, medically trained source before making any drastic changes to your diet or health regimen, especially based on one news story or study.

Where Can I Find Reliable Information on Weight-Loss Programs, Diets, and Organizations?

Self-Directed Education

The Obesity Prevention Source, offered through Harvard University's T.H. Chan School of Public Health, provides a comprehensive overview of obesity prevention guidelines, including a "Healthy Weight Checklist."

The Obesity Action Coalition (OAC) is a nonprofit advocacy and education organization that seeks to empower people with obesity and those who desire weight loss by providing a variety of educational resources; these include the following:

- Brochures. Most notably *Understanding Your Weight Loss Options*, which summarizes a wide list of available weight-loss tools.

- http://www.obesityaction.org/educational-resources/brochures-and-guides/understanding-your-weight-loss-options-brochure.

- Webinars. OAC offers a FREE educational webinar series that addresses topics such as "*Does that really work? Deciphering popular weight loss trends*" and "*Who's in control? The science behind willpower.*" (http://www.obesityaction.org/educational-resources/oac-educational-webinars)

  The Obesity Society (TOS) seeks to "Better understand, prevent, and treat obesity to improve the lives of those affected through research, education, and advocacy." (Obesity Society, 2017). In addition to partnering with the OAC to provide the aforementioned resources, TOS has expertly written patient resources that include handouts such as "Medications for weight loss" (Rubino, 2017) and "How much weight do I need to lose?" (Saunders, 2017).

Time to Act on Obesity is a program developed to help improve obesity education. In addition to patient handouts, it contains free obesity training modules written by obesity experts at Harvard University and the Massachusetts Institute of Technology. The program is sponsored by Ethicon.

Obesity Specialists

As you have read in the previous chapters in *Facing Overweight and Obesity*, obesity management is complex and requires a comprehensive care plan. Not only is it okay to ask for help on your weight-management journey, it's often essential for successful weight loss and maintenance. Figure 17-2 summarizes the most common obesity specialists who assist with weight loss.

Specialist Type	Potential Role in Obesity Management	How to Locate a Specialist/ Center of Excellence
Mental Health Provider • Bariatric Counselors • Bariatric Educators • Psychologists	Focus on managing the behavioral and psychological aspects of obesity management (Walters, 2017). They can help you figure out *"why"* you eat which is essential for achieving lasting weight loss.	**American Association of Bariatric Counselors** http://nabc-certification.org/blog/ **American Psychological Association** http://www.apa.org/helpcenter/weight-control.pdf
Nutrition Support • Nutritionist • Dietician	Proper nutrition is essential to weight loss and weight maintenance. Both nutritionists and dieticians can assist in identifying eating patterns contributing to obesity and creating an individualized weight loss eating plan. Dieticians have typically more training than nutritionist and are certified through the Commission on Dietetic Registration (CDR) which now offers obesity specialization.	**Certification for Dietetic Registration Board** **Certified Specialist in Obesity and Weight Management** https://www.cdrnet.org/interdisciplinary -Click "Board Certified...By State"
Physicians, NP, PA & Allied Health Professionals	Clinicians trained in obesity medicine seek to provide comprehensive obesity management that includes lifestyle optimization, medication management and referral to appropriate bariatric endoscopic or surgical interventions when needed. Certifications for allied professionals is offered through The Obesity Medicine Association. The American Board of Obesity Medicine provides certification to obesity medicine physicians (bariatricians).	**The American Board of Obesity Medicine** https://abom.learningbuilder.com/public/membersearch **The Obesity Medicine Association** https://obesitymedicine.org/find-obesity-treatment/ **The Obesity Society** http://www.obesity.org/resources/clinician-directory
Surgeons, Bariatric	Bariatric surgeons specialize in surgical procedures aimed at treating obesity such as gastric bypass surgery. Many work in Bariatric Centers of Excellence (**MBSAQIP**) which provide high quality interdisciplinary patient care before & after surgery to ensure successful surgical outcomes	**American Society for Bariatric and Metabolic Surgeons** https://asmbs.org/patients/find-a-provider **Metabolic and Bariatric Surgery Accreditation and Quality Improvement Program (MBSAQIP)** https://www.facs.org/search/bariatric-surgery-centers

Figure 17-2: Specialist resources for weight loss.

What Internet Sites Can I Use to Learn More About Obesity?

There are several organizations and institutions committed to offering high-quality obesity information. Some of them have already been listed in the preceding sections.

Figure 17-3 summarizes these organizations and institutions. You can use it as a quick reference guide for finding obesity resources.

Obesity Focused Professional Organizations		
The Obesity Society	Unites various sectors of obesity care-clinicians, researchers, educators & policy makers to better prevent & treat obesity. Patient & professional resources available for free on website.	Homepage: http://www.obesity.org/home Infographics: http://www.obesity.org/resources/facts-about-obesity/infographics
Obesity Medicine Association	Strives to advance the field of obesity medicine. This website provides patient education and professional resources.	Homepage: https://obesitymedicine.org
Obesity Action Coalition	Utilizes advocacy, education, and support to empower individuals with obesity to better health. Provides education, health initiatives and weight support groups.	Homepage: http://www.obesityaction.org
American Society for Metabolic and Bariatric Surgery	A society for surgeons and bariatric providers dedicated to the surgical management of obesity. Patient information videos and professional resources available	Homepage: https://asmbs.org
American Board of Obesity Medicine	Provides standardized obesity board certification for physicians. This site is to useful to find qualified obesity specialists.	Homepage: www.abom.org
Government Organizations		
Center Disease Control Overweight & Obesity	Provides obesity data, statistics as well as educational resources and population health strategies for decreasing obesity.	Homepage: https://www.cdc.gov/obesity/
National Heart, Lung and Blood Institute: Obesity	Provides information for determining your obesity risk, education and research participation opportunities.	Homepage: https://www.nhlbi.nih.gov/health/health-topics/topics/obe
World Health Organization	International obesity data and tool for education and community planning provided.	Homepage: http://www.who.int/topics/obesity/en/
Obesity Advocacy (Collaborative Efforts)		
Campaign to End Obesity	Works with leaders across industry, academia and public health with policymakers and their advisors to fill the unmet gaps in obesity policy	Homepage: http://obesitycampaign.org
National Alliance for Nutrition and Activity	Aims to reduce illness, disabilities and death caused by diet and inactivity related diseases through policy and advocacy.	Homepage: https://cspinet.org/national-alliance-nutrition-and-activity
Obesity Care Advocacy Network	Seeks to align key obesity stakeholders and the obesity community to advance obesity education, legislative efforts & policy.	Homepage: http://www.obesitycareadvocacynetwork.com/
Free Online Course/ Resource		
Time to Act on Obesity	Provides self paced obesity courses and patient handouts developed by obesity specialists from Harvard University and Massachusetts Institute of Technology.	Homepage: https://www.timetoactonobesity.org/

Figure 17-3: Organizations and institutions with obesity resources.

Conclusion

Although, it can be difficult to navigate the sea of weight-management information, this chapter has provided you high-quality, evidence-based, obesity-related resources. You have been empowered with tools that you'll need to determine high-quality information as you continue your quest for knowledge about obesity.

GLOSSARY

Abdominal fat: The type of fat that surrounds your internal organs and appears to give you a "beer belly"; it is a predictor of heart disease, type 2 diabetes, insulin resistance, and some cancers.

Acid-alkaline diet: A diet that is based on the premise that by helping your body control your pH through diet, you'll gain health and longevity.

Adipose tissue: Body fat.

Alpha-melanocyte stimulating hormone: An endogenous peptide hormone and neuropeptide of the melanocortin family. It is responsible for pigmentation primarily of the hair and skin and it plays a role in feeding behavior, energy homeostasis, sexual activity, and protection against ischemia and reperfusion injury.

Alstrom syndrome: An autosomal recessive syndrome with retinitis pigmentosa, nystagmus, and early loss of central vision, deafness, obesity, and diabetes.

American College of Sports Medicine: A professional society that promotes and integrates scientific research, education, and practical applications of sports medicine.

American Heart Association: A nonprofit organization designed to improve care for people with heart disease.

Amphetamine: A stimulant drug that can be abused.

Anesthesia: The temporary loss of consciousness and sensation that is commonly used as a part of surgery.

Angiotensin II receptor-blocking (ARB) agent: A medication used to treat high blood pressure. It works by blocking the site of action of angiotensin II, which typically functions to constrict blood vessels and increase blood pressure.

Angiotensin-converting enzyme (ACE) inhibitor: A medication used to treat high blood pressure. It works by blocking the conversion of angiotensin I to angiotensin II, thereby reducing the pressure in the blood vessels.

Anhedonia: A lack of interest or pleasure in almost all activities.

Anorexia nervosa: An eating disorder that involves a believe that one has excess weight.

Anthropomorphic measurements: Metrics that are used to assess the size, shape, and composition of the human body.

Anti-coagulation: The process of slowing down the body's ability to make blood clots. It is accomplished via use of medications known as anti-coagulants (that are often used by those who suffer from coronary artery disease, thromboembolic disease, or strokes).

Anti-inflammatory agents: Medications that help to reduce swelling or inflammation.

Antioxidant: One of many widely used synthetic or natural substances that prevent or delay deterioration by the action of oxygen.

Aplastic anemia: A rare disease in which the bone marrow and the hematopoietic stem cells that reside there are damaged. This causes a deficiency of all three blood cell types (pancytopenia): red blood cells (anemia), white blood cells (leukopenia), and platelets (thrombocytopenia).

Apnea: The sudden stopping of breathing; an involuntary action.

Apolipoproteins: Proteins that bind lipids (oil-soluble substances such as fat and cholesterol) to form lipoproteins; they transport lipids through the lymphatic and circulatory systems.

Arrhythmia: An abnormal heart rhythm.

Arteries: Part of the circulatory system that delivers oxygenated blood from the heart to the rest of the body.

Arthritis: A generic term that refers to any medical condition (e.g., osteoarthritis) that affects the joints.

Ataxia: A condition with impaired coordination.

Atkins diet: A low-carbohydrate diet program used to achieve weight loss.

Autosomal dominant: In an autosomal dominant disease, if you inherit the abnormal gene from only one parent, you can get the disease.

Autosomal recessive: In an autosomal recessive disorder, two copies of an abnormal gene must be present for the disease or trait to develop.

Bardet-Biedl syndrome: An autosomal recessive disorder characterized by intellectual disability, pigmentary retinopathy, obesity, polydactyly, and hypogonadism.

Bariatric surgery: Weight-loss surgery; for example, Roux-en-Y gastric bypass, gastric sleeve, adjustable gastric band, and bilio-pancreatic diversion with duodenal switch.

Barrett's esophagus: A condition that develops due to long-term exposure to stomach acid, often associated with gastroesophageal reflux disease (GERD). In this condition, the normal tissue of the esophagus begins to be replaced by tissue that resembles the intestinal lining. This condition can increase the risk of developing esophageal cancer.

Behaviorists: Practitioners who apply a systematic approach to understanding the behavior of humans and other animals. They assume that all behaviors are either reflexes produced by a response to certain stimuli in the environment, or a consequence of that individual's history, including especially reinforcement and punishment.

Benzphetamine: A substituted amphetamine used short term along with a doctor-approved, reduced-calorie diet, exercise, and behavioral program for weight loss. It is prescribed for obesity in individuals who have been unable to lose weight through exercise and dieting alone.

Beta endorphins: Endogenous opioid neuropeptides and peptide hormones that are produced in the pituitary gland that are powerful pain suppressors.

Biliopancreatic diversion: A surgical procedure (in which part of the stomach is removed) that restricts food intake and the number of calories and amount of nutrients that the body can absorb.

Bioelectrical impedance analysis (BIA): A method of assessing your body composition, the measurement of body fat in relation to lean body mass.

BiPAP: An abbreviation for bilevel positive airway pressures, which is a non-invasive type of ventilation that has two pressure settings, one for inhalation and one for exhalation.

Bipolar disorder: A mood disorder characterized by manic and depressive episodes.

Black-box warning: This is the strictest warning put in the labeling of prescription drugs or drug products by the US Food and Drug Administration (FDA) when there is reasonable evidence of an association of a serious hazard with the drug.

Blinding: A process to avoid bias during clinical trials by being unaware of which drug (e.g., placebo or active drug) is being received by the participant (and potentially by the examiner).

Blood glucose level: The level of blood sugar in the blood.

Blood urea nitrogen (BUN): A medical test that measures the amount of urea nitrogen found in blood. It is a measure of kidney function.

Blood–brain barrier: A highly selective semipermeable membrane barrier that separates the circulating blood from the brain and extracellular fluid in the central nervous system (CNS).

Body image: How one views one's sense of self.

Body mass index (BMI): A number derived from your height and weight that indicates your weight classification.

Bowel obstruction: Also known as intestinal obstruction, it is a mechanical or functional obstruction of the intestines that prevents the normal movement of the products of digestion.

Bradycardia: Abnormally slow heart rates.

Bupropion: An antidepressant drug that has also helped people to stop smoking.

Cabbage soup diet: A low-fat, high-fiber diet that consists of a fat-free cabbage soup that is eaten one to three times a day.

Calcium channel: An ion channel that shows selective permeability to calcium ions. It is sometimes synonymous with voltage-gated calcium channel, although there are also ligand-gated calcium channels.

Caliper: A device used to measure the distance between opposite sides of an object.

Camellia sinensis: A species of evergreen shrub or small tree whose leaves and leaf buds are used to produce tea.

Carbonic anhydrase inhibitors: A class of pharmaceuticals that suppress the activity of carbonic anhydrase. Their clinical use has been established as anti-glaucoma agents, diuretics, anti-epileptics, in the management of mountain sickness, gastric and duodenal ulcers, idiopathic intracranial hypertension, neurological disorders, or osteoporosis.

Cardiac catheterization: A procedure used to diagnose and treat heart disease. It involves inserting a catheter into the heart through blood vessels to check for blood flow or blockage.

Cardiac ischemia: The name for decreased blood flow and oxygen to the heart muscle.

Case manager: Registered nurses (RNs) who develop, implement, and evaluate individualized patient care plans. Case managers act as social workers, advocate patient welfare, and serve as a liaison between patients, their families, and health-care providers.

Centers for Disease Control and Prevention (CDC): A public health agency in the United States that aims to prevent and control disease.

Central nervous system (CNS): Nerves originating in the brain and the spinal cord.

Central sleep apnea: A condition in which your breathing stops on its own (because your brain doesn't send proper signals to the muscles that control breathing).

Cerebrovascular accident (CVA): The medical term for stroke. It occurs when blood flow suddenly stops to a certain part of the brain.

Cerebrovascular disease: Any condition that affects the blood vessels of the brain and its circulation.

Cholecystectomy: A surgical procedure in which the gallbladder is removed.

Cholecystitis: An inflammation of the gallbladder.

Cholelithiasis: The medical term for gallstone disease.

Cholesterol: A pearly, fat-like steroid alcohol found in animal fats and oils that can clog your arteries with plaque buildup and lead to strokes or heart attacks.

Cholycystokinin: A hormone that is secreted by cells in the duodenum and stimulates the release of bile into the intestine and the secretion of enzymes by the pancreas.

Chromium picolinate: A chemical compound that's sometimes used as an alternative therapy or as a nutritional supplement.

Chromosomes: Structures in the nucleus of cells that transmit genetic information.

Circulatory system: Also known as the cardiovascular system. It is responsible for the circulation of blood as well as a variety of nutrients, proteins, and hormones to different parts of the body.

Cirrhosis: A complication of scarring/fibrosis in the liver due to liver disease that occurs over time.

Clinical research trial: A research study that evaluates new ways to prevent, detect, or treat a condition.

Cognitive-behavioral therapy (CBT): A type of psychotherapy that focuses on how to change thoughts and behaviors.

Colonoscopy: A procedure to visually inspect the inside of the colon (i.e., large intestine).

Co-morbidity: Co-occurrence of more than one disease at the same time in an individual.

Complementary and alternative medicine: Medical products and practices that are not part of standard medical care. These practices include massage, acupuncture, tai chi, and drinking green tea.

Complete blood count (CBC): A laboratory test that assesses white blood cells, red blood cells, and platelets in the bloodstream.

Congestive heart failure: A condition in which the heart is unable to pump blood effectively.

Continuous positive airway pressure (CPAP): Like BiPAP, a non-invasive form of ventilation. However, it has only one pressure setting and the pressure is delivered in a continuous form throughout the breathing cycle.

Coronary arteries: The arteries that supply blood to the heart.

Coronary artery disease (CAD): Narrowing of the coronary arteries (the arteries that supply the heart muscle with oxygen and nutrients) caused by buildup of plaque. This is the most common form of heart disease in the United States.

Cortisol: A steroid hormone, in the glucocorticoid class of hormones. This is a stress hormone.

C-reactive protein: An acute-phase protein of hepatic origin found in blood plasma, whose levels rise in response to inflammation (following interleukin-6 secretion by macrophages and T cells).

Creatinine: A compound that is produced by metabolism of creatine and excreted in the urine; it is a measure of kidney functions.

Cytokines: Non-antibody proteins released when in contact with specific antigens, which act as intercellular mediators, generating an immune response.

Deep vein thrombosis (DVT): The condition in which a blood clot forms in the "deep veins" of the body, usually the legs.

Deoxyribonucleic acid (DNA): A nucleic acid that constitutes the genetic material of all cellular organisms.

Diabetes: A chronic disorder marked by elevated levels of blood glucose caused by not being able to make enough insulin.

Diastolic blood pressure: The number on the bottom of a blood pressure reading that refers to the blood pressure when your heart is between beats.

Diethylpropion: A stimulant like amphetamine; it is an appetite suppressant that affects the central nervous system.

Distal gastric bypass: A procedure that is usually performed for patients who are in the super obese group (BMI more than 50). Additional small intestine is bypassed so there will be less intestinal surface for absorption of calories, especially fat. This results in more frequent bowel movements per day.

Double-blind, placebo-controlled studies: A type of experiment in which neither the patients/subjects nor the experimenters are told which drug is being administered (so as to limit their bias influencing the results of the experiment).

Dual energy X-ray absorptometry (DEXA or DXA) scan: A means of measuring bone density.

Dumping syndrome: A complex reaction thought to be due to excessively rapid emptying of the gastric contents into the jejunum, manifest by nausea, weakness, sweating, and diarrhea after ingestion of food.

Duodenal switch: A weight-loss surgery, also known as biliopancreatic diversion with duodenal switch, or gastric reduction.

Dysmorphic feature: A difference of body structure that can be mild or severe (e.g., a congenital heart defect).

Dysthymia: Low-level depression or sadness lasting for a year or more.

Echocardiogram: Also known as a cardiac ultrasound, it is used for the diagnosis and management of heart disease.

Electrocardiogram (EKG/ECG): A test that records the electrical activity of the heart.

Electrolytes: Includes substances (such as sodium, potassium, magnesium, and phosphate) that are found in the human body. Electrolytes help with cellular function and stability.

Emotional eating: Eating that occurs in response to an emotion and occurs without being hungry.

Endocrine organ: A gland (e.g., pituitary, thyroid, adrenals, ovaries, testes) that is part of the endocrine system that carries hormones into the circulatory system to distant target organs.

Endocrinologist: A physician who specializes in the diagnosis and treatment of those with endocrine, hormonal, or glandular problem.

Endometrial cancer: A type of cancer that affects the lining of the uterus.

Endorphins: Neuropeptides that bind to opioid receptors and that have analgesic effects.

Endoscopy: Also known as esophagogastroduodenoscopy (EGD). This is a procedure in which an endoscope is inserted into the esophagus to obtain a better view of the lining of the esophagus, stomach, and intestine.

Environmental factors: Factors (e.g., soil, water, climate) that influence living organisms.

Esophagus: A part of the body that connects the throat to the stomach.

Exclusion criteria: A list of criteria that precludes entry into a research study.

Exercise specialists: Fitness trainers or instructors who create exercise plans designed to improve health for clients, such as those at high risk for heart, metabolic, or lung disease.

Explicit weight bias: Explicit biases are intentional and conscious and are assessed using self-report measures.

False positive: A test result that incorrectly indicates that a particular condition or attribute is present.

Fasting blood sugar: The blood glucose level obtained after not having eaten (for example, first thing in the morning after waking up).

Fasting glucose: A fasting glucose test is a measure of blood glucose levels after a person fasts for at least 8 hours.

Fat-free mass: Also called Lean Body Mass (LBM), this is the total amount of non-fat (lean) parts of the body. It typically consists of approximately 73% water, 20% protein, 6% mineral, and 1% ash.

Fatty liver disease: A condition in which fat builds up in your liver.

Fecal incontinence: Also called bowel incontinence, the inability to control bowel movements, causing stool (feces) to leak unexpectedly from the rectum; it ranges from an occasional leakage of stool while passing gas to a complete loss of bowel control.

Fecal urgency: Urgency occurs when the arrival of feces in the rectum causes strong contractions and precipitates anal relaxation, giving the feeling that passage of stool is about to occur.

Feedback loop: Feedback occurs when outputs of a system are routed back as inputs as part of a chain that forms a circuit or loop.

Fellowship: An advanced clinical training program that occurs after residency for physicians in the United States. Disciplines that have clinical fellowships include Cardiology, Gastroenterology, Pulmonology, and Endocrinology.

Fluoxetine: Also known by the trade names Prozac and Sarafem among others, it is an antidepressant of the selective serotonin re-uptake inhibitor (SSRI) class. It is used for the treatment of major depressive disorder (MDD), obsessive–compulsive disorder (OCD), bulimia nervosa, panic disorder, and premenstrual dysphoric disorder.

Food and Drug Administration (FDA): A government agency that assesses the safety and efficacy of medications, and approves them for use.

FTO gene: The *FTO* gene located on chromosome 16, encodes the fat mass and obesity-associated protein, also known as alpha-ketoglutarate-dependent dioxygenase. Certain variants of the *FTO* gene appear to be correlated with obesity in humans.

Gallstones: Hardened deposits of digestive fluid that form in your gallbladder (a small organ on the right side of your abdomen just beneath your liver).

Gamma amino butyric acid (GABA): GABA is a neurotransmitter that sends chemical messages through the brain and the nervous system and is involved in regulating communication between brain cells. The role of GABA is to inhibit or reduce the activity of the neurons or nerve cells.

Garancii cambogia: A tropical fruit, also known as the Malabar tamarind, that is used as a popular weight-loss supplement thought to reduce the body's ability to make fat and to "put the brakes" on your appetite.

Gastric balloon: A soft silicon balloon that is inserted into your stomach. The balloon partially fills the stomach, which leads to a feeling of fullness.

Gastroesophageal reflux disease (GERD): A condition in which stomach acid regurgitates backward into the esophagus, leading to irritation of the esophagus lining.

Generic: A consumer product having no brand name or registered trademark.

Genes: The structures within a cell's nucleus into which deoxyribonucleic acid (DNA) is packed; many genes form a chromosome and encode the "blueprints" for a cell's function.

Genetic Information Non-Discrimination Act (GINA): A federal law that protects individuals from genetic discrimination in health insurance and employment. Genetic discrimination is the misuse of genetic information.

Genetic predisposition: An increased likelihood of developing a particular disease based on a person's genetic makeup.

Genetic variability: This is a measure of the tendency of individual genotypes in a population to vary from one another. Variability is different from genetic diversity, which is the amount of variation seen in a particular population.

Genetic variation: A term used to describe the variation in the DNA sequence in each of our genomes, which occurs within and among populations.

Genetics: The study of genes and hereditary variation.

Genotype: The part of the genetic makeup of a cell (and an individual) that determines one of its characteristics.

Ghrelin: The "hunger hormone"; a peptide hormone that stimulates appetite, increases food intake, and promotes fat storage.

Glucagon-like peptide (GLP-1): A 30-amino-acid-long peptide hormone derived from the tissue-specific post-translational processing of the proglucagon gene. It is produced and secreted by intestinal enteroendocrine L-cells and certain neurons within the nucleus of the solitary tract in the brainstem upon food consumption.

Glucose: Simple sugar molecule used by the body for energy.

Glucose intolerance: A pre-diabetic state of hyperglycemia that is associated with insulin resistance and an increased risk of cardiovascular disease.

Glycemic-index diet: This usually refers to a specific diet plan that uses the index as the primary or only guide for meal planning. Unlike some other plans, a glycemic-index diet doesn't necessarily specify portion sizes or the optimal number of calories, carbohydrates, or fats for weight loss or weight maintenance.

Glycogen: Stored glucose.

"Gold standard": Best approach.

Gout: A condition in which the body is unable to metabolize uric acid appropriately, leading to uric acid deposits in the joints and thus causing pain and/or inflammation.

Gout attacks: The sudden onset of pain in a gout-affected joint. It is often characterized by redness, swelling, warmth, and sensitivity to touch of the affected joint.

Group therapy: Psychotherapy done with multiple individuals and led by a therapist.

Heart attack: A condition that occurs when blood flow to the heart is blocked.

Heart failure: *See* congestive heart failure.

Heartburn: A burning sensation in the chest, usually due to acid reflux.

Heat stroke: A condition marked by fever and often by unconsciousness, caused by failure of the body's temperature-regulating mechanism when exposed to excessively high temperatures.

Helicobacter pylori: Previously known as *Campylobacter pylori*, this is a gram-negative, microaerophilic bacterium usually found in the stomach; it is present in people with chronic gastritis and gastric ulcers, conditions not previously believed to have a microbial cause. It is also linked to the development of duodenal ulcers and stomach cancer.

Hematocrit: A measurement of the proportion of red blood cells in your blood to the total blood volume.

Hemoglobin: A protein within red blood cells that carries oxygen from the lungs to the tissues of the body, and carbon dioxide from tissues back to the lungs.

Hemoglobin AIC: Glycated hemoglobin (also known as HbA1c); a blood test that measures your average blood sugar level over the prior three months by measuring the amount of glucose that is attached to red blood cells.

Hepatobiliary (HIDA) scan: An imaging study used to diagnose conditions related to the liver, gallbladder, and bile ducts.

Hepatotoxicity: Derived from hepatic toxicity, it implies chemical-driven liver damage. Drug-induced liver injury is a cause of acute and chronic liver disease.

Hereditary: Determined by genetic factors and therefore able to be passed on from parents to their offspring or descendants.

Heterozygous: Having dissimilar pairs of genes for any hereditary characteristic.

High-density lipoprotein (HDL): A protein commonly referred to as "good cholesterol." HDL removes "bad cholesterol" from the bloodstream and it decreases your risk of heart disease.

Histamine (H2) blocker: A class of medications that blocks the action of histamine, specifically at the H_2 receptor, in the stomach.

Homeostasis: The stable condition of an organism and of its internal environment, the maintenance or regulation of the stable condition, or its equilibrium; the balance of bodily functions.

Homicidal ideation: Thoughts about homicide, which range from vague ideas of revenge to detailed and fully formulated plans without the act itself.

Homozygous: Having identical pairs of genes for any given pair of hereditary characteristics.

Hoodia gordonii: Also known as Bushman's hat, is a leafless spiny succulent plant that is supposed to have therapeutic properties in folk medicine.

Hormone: A substance produced by glands that plays a role in cell signaling and physiologic regulation.

Hyperammonemic encephalopathy: Increased entry of ammonia to the brain is a primary cause of neurological disorders associated with hyperammonemia, such as congenital deficiencies of urea cycle enzymes, hepatic encephalopathies, Reye syndrome, several other metabolic disorders, and some toxic encephalopathies.

Hyperglycemia: An elevated blood glucose level.

Hyperlipidemia: A high amount of fat particles (lipids) such as cholesterol and triglycerides in the blood.

Hyperprolactinemia: The presence of abnormally high levels of prolactin in the blood.

Hypertension: High blood pressure.

Hyperthermia: The condition of having a body temperature greatly above normal.

Hypoglycemia: Low blood sugar.

Hypomania: A mild form of mania, marked by elation and hyperactivity.

Hyponatremia: A condition that occurs when the level of sodium in your blood is abnormally low.

Hypothalamus: A portion of the brain that contains several small nuclei with a variety of functions. One of the most important functions of the hypothalamus is to link the nervous system to the endocrine system via the pituitary gland (hypophysis).

Hypothesis: A supposition that appears to explain a group of phenomena and is advanced as a basis for further investigation.

Hypothyroidism: A condition involving an under-active thyroid gland.

Hypoventilation syndrome: A generic name for a variety of conditions that cause inadequate ventilation (gas exchange between oxygen and carbon dioxide). Obesity hypoventilation syndrome is an example.

Hypoxia: A state caused by a less-than-adequate amount of oxygen being delivered to tissues.

Idiopathic intracranial hypertension: Increased pressure within the brain of uncertain etiology.

Implicit weight bias: Implicit biases are automatically activated, can occur unconsciously, and are typically measured using response-latency tasks, like the Implicit Association Task (IAT), which measure the strength of association between social categories and attitudes.

Inclusion criteria: A list of criteria required of participants before they can be included in a study.

Individual therapy: One-on-one psychotherapy led by a therapist.

Inflammation: A condition in which part of the body becomes swollen, red, warm, and painful. Inflammation is a natural part of the body's immune response.

Informed consent: A process by which potential participants are provided with information about a study as well as its risks and benefits, enabling a participant to freely enroll or refuse to participate.

Inherited: Derived (a quality, characteristic, or predisposition) genetically from one's parents or ancestors.

Insulin: A protein produced by the pancreas that lowers blood glucose levels by promoting energy storage in the body's tissues.

Insulin resistance: A condition in which the cells fail to respond to the hormone insulin. This results in a high blood sugar level.

Intellectual disability: A disability characterized by significant limitations in intellectual function (or IQ) and behavior; previously called mental retardation.

Intra-gastric balloon: A newer kind of weight-loss procedure involving placement of a saline-filled silicone balloon in your stomach, leading to feeling fuller faster; it helps with weight loss by limiting how much you can eat.

Jaundice: Yellowing of a person, caused by elevated levels of bilirubin.

Jenny Craig diet: A weight-loss program that offers consultations, pre-packed foods, and motivation to support users. It claims to be an all-encompassing weight-loss solution that can promote real change.

Kidney function: A measure of how well your kidneys are working. Often ascertained through a creatinine and blood urea nitrogen (BUN) tests.

Kidney function tests: To check for kidney disease, health-care providers use a blood test that checks how well your kidneys are filtering your blood, called glomerular filtration rate (GFR), and a urine test to check for albumin (a protein that can pass into the urine when the kidneys are damaged).

Kidney stones: Also known as renal lithiasis or nephrolithiasis, these are hard deposits made of minerals and salts that form inside your kidneys. Kidney stones have many causes.

Laparoscopy: A surgical procedure in which a fiber-optic instrument is inserted through the abdominal wall to view the organs in the abdomen or to permit a surgical procedure.

Lap band: A lap band is an inflatable silicone device placed around the top portion of the stomach to treat obesity, intended to slow consumption of food and thus reduce the amount of food consumed.

Leptin: The hormone of energy expenditure, predominantly made by adipose cells that helps to regulate hunger by inhibiting hunger.

Leptin receptor deficiency: A condition that causes severe obesity beginning in the first few months of life. Affected individuals are of normal weight at birth, but they are constantly hungry and quickly gain weight. The extreme hunger leads to chronic excessive eating (hyperphagia) and obesity.

Libido: Sex drive; sexual appetite.

Lipase: A pancreatic enzyme that catalyzes the breakdown of fats to fatty acids and glycerol or other alcohols.

Lipid profile: Measurement of various lipids/fatty substances in your blood.

Liraglutide: A derivative of human incretin (metabolic hormone) glucagon-like peptide-1 (GLP-1) that is used as a long-acting glucagon-like peptide-1 receptor agonist, binding to the same receptors as does the endogenous metabolic hormone GLP-1 that stimulates insulin secretion.

Liver: An organ located in the upper-right quadrant of the abdomen, below the diaphragm. Its roles in metabolism include the regulation of glycogen storage, decomposition of red blood cells, and the production of hormones.

Liver biopsy: A test done to aid in the diagnosis of liver disease. It involves inserting a small needle through your skin and into the liver.

Liver function tests: Blood tests that assess the function of your liver, via measurement of various components.

Liver toxicity: Implies chemical-driven liver damage. Drug-induced liver injury is a cause of acute and chronic liver disease. The liver plays a central role in transforming and clearing chemicals and is susceptible to the toxicity from these agents.

Liver transplantation: The replacement of a diseased part of the liver with a healthy liver from another person.

Lorcaserin: A weight-loss drug; it reduces appetite by activating a type of serotonin receptor, known as the 5-HT_{2C} receptor, in a region of the brain called the hypothalamus, which is known to control appetite.

Low-Density Lipoprotein (LDL): This is the "bad cholesterol." It collects around the walls of blood vessels, leading to their narrowing, and causing blockages.

Macrobiotic diet: This diet involves eating brown rice and other whole grains (such as barley, millet, oats, quinoa, spelt, rye, and teff) in which yin and yang are closest to being in balance.

Major depressive disorder (MDD): A disorder in which individuals experience a depressed mood, sleep disruption, lack of or increase in appetite, feelings of guilt, decreased concentration, psychomotor agitation or retardation, and suicidal thoughts.

Mania: A mental illness marked by periods of great excitement, euphoria, delusions, and overactivity.

Megaloblastic anemia: An anemia characterized by many large immature and dysfunctional red blood cells (megaloblasts) in the bone marrow and also by hypersegmented neutrophils (those exhibiting five or more nuclear lobes ["segments"]).

Melanocortin-4 receptor (MC-4R): A protein that in humans is encoded by the *MC4R* gene. It encodes the MC_4 protein, which is involved in feeding behavior.

Melanocortin-4 receptor deficiency (MC-4R): A condition in which there is a deficiency of melanocortin-4 receptors.

Mesocorticolimbic dopamine system: Sometimes referred to as the reward pathway, this is a dopaminergic pathway in the brain.

Mesolimbic reward system: The mesolimbic pathway, sometimes referred to as the reward pathway, is a dopaminergic pathway in the brain.

Meta-analysis: Uses a statistical approach to combine the results from multiple studies in an effort to increase power (over individual studies), improve estimates of the size of the effect and/or to resolve uncertainty when reports disagree.

Metabolic acidosis: A condition that occurs when the body produces excessive quantities of acid or when the kidneys are not removing enough acid from the body.

Metabolic syndrome: A cluster of conditions in which there is an increased risk of heart disease, stroke, and diabetes. There are five parameters that are looked at when diagnosing metabolic syndrome: abdominal obesity, high blood pressure, high blood sugar, high triglycerides, and low levels of HDL ("good cholesterol").

Metabolites: Break-down products of chemical reactions.

Metformin: A first-line medication to prevent or treat people with type 2 diabetes.

Mg/dL: Milligrams per deciliter. It is the standard unit of measurement for blood glucose levels.

Mindfulness: Being present in the moment, paying attention to bodily sensations and experiences.

Minimally invasive surgery: In minimally invasive surgery, doctors use a variety of techniques to operate with less damage to the body than with open surgery. In general, minimally invasive surgery is associated with less pain, a shorter hospital stay, and fewer complications.

Mixed sleep apnea: A type of sleep apnea in which both obstructive sleep apnea and central sleep apnea are present.

Mm Hg: Millimeters of mercury. It is the standard unit of measurement for blood pressure.

Mnemonic: An association that helps us remember something.

Molecules: A group of atoms bonded together, representing the smallest fundamental unit of a chemical compound that can take part in a chemical reaction.

Mu opioid antagonist: A receptor antagonist that acts on one of the opioid receptors.

Multi-disciplinary care: Care provided by providers from several disciplines in a collaborative manner.

Mutation: The changing structure of a gene, resulting in a variant form that may be transmitted to subsequent generations, caused by the alteration of single base units of DNA or the deletion, insertion, or rearrangement of larger sections of genes or chromosomes.

Myocardial infarction (MI): A heart attack; sudden damage to the heart caused by a clot in an artery that supplies blood to the heart muscle.

NASH: Also known as non-alcoholic steatohepatitis. This is a liver disease that is not related to alcohol use. Those with NASH have fat in their livers that causes inflammation and cirrhosis.

Nephrotoxicity: Toxicity in the kidneys. It is a poisonous effect of some substances, both toxic chemicals and medications, on renal function. There are various forms, and some drugs can affect renal function in more than one way. Nephrotoxins are substances displaying nephrotoxicity.

Neurochemical: A small organic molecule or peptide that participates in neural activity.

Neuropsychiatric symptoms: These most often include depression, psychosis, apathy, hyperactivity/agitation, sleep disorders, and prefrontal syndromes.

Neurotransmitter: A chemical substance that is released at the end of a nerve fiber by the arrival of a nerve impulse and, by diffusing across the synapse or junction, causes the transfer of the impulse to another nerve fiber, a muscle fiber, or some other structure.

Nicotine: A potent parasympathomimetic stimulant and an alkaloid found in the nightshade family of plants; often found in the smoke of tobacco products, which can lead to insulin sensitivity, insulin resistance, an increased risk of developing metabolic syndrome, type 2 diabetes, and cardiovascular disease.

Non-alcoholic fatty liver disease (NAFLD): Like NASH, this condition is not related to alcohol use. Fat accumulates in the liver. NASH is a type of NAFLD.

Norepinephrine-dopamine re-uptake inhibitor (NDRI): A drug that acts as a re-uptake inhibitor for the neurotransmitters norepinephrine (NE) and dopamine (DA) by blocking the action of the NE transporter (NET) and the DA transporter (DAT), respectively.

Nucleus accumbens: A region in the basal forebrain rostral to the preoptic area of the hypothalamus. It has a significant role in addiction.

Nutraceutical: A food containing health-giving additives and having medicinal benefit.

Nutrisystem diet: Nutrisystem aims to simplify weight loss, removing the decisions about which foods will fit your diet or counting calories or carbs (because you buy most of your food from Nutrisystem).

Nutritionists: A person who studies or is an expert in nutrition. A registered dietitian nutritionist is the recognized health-care expert in the field of nutrition.

Obesity: Defined medically as having a body mass index of greater than or equal to 30 kg/m^2.

Obesity hypoventilation syndrome: A condition seen in overweight individuals that leads to inadequate breathing, low oxygen levels, and high carbon dioxide levels in the blood.

Obesity medicine: A discipline that focuses on the prevention and treatment of obesity.

Obesity medicine specialist: A physician who specializes in the comprehensive care of people with overweight or obesity.

Obesogenic: Tending to cause obesity.

Obstructive sleep apnea (OSA): A type of sleep apnea that is caused by obstructions in the upper airway. It is the most common form of sleep apnea.

Opioids: A class of drugs that include the illegal drug heroin, synthetic opioids, such as fentanyl, and pain relievers available legally by prescription, such as oxycodone (OxyContin), hydrocodone (Vicodin), codeine, morphine, and many others. These drugs are chemically related and interact with opioid receptors on nerve cells in the body and brain.

Ornish diet: This diet involves eating all the beans, legumes, fruits, grains, and vegetables you need to feel full, and eating low- or non-fat dairy products, such as milk, cheese, and yogurt, in moderation. Only 10 percent of calories should come from fat.

Osteoarthritis (OA): A type of arthritis that occurs secondary to "wear and tear" of joints due to the breakdown of cartilage in the joints. It leads to bone damage.

Osteoporosis: A disease that thins and weakens the bones. Your bones become fragile and break easily, especially the bones in the hip, spine, and wrist.

Overeaters Anonymous (OA): A support group for binge eating.

Overweight: Above a weight considered normal or desirable.

Oxylate nephropathy: Characterized by tubular crystalline deposits of calcium oxalate leading to acute and chronic tubular injury, interstitial fibrosis, and progressive renal insufficiency.

Pain specialist: Health-care specialists who focus on the diagnosis and management of chronic pain.

Paleo diet: A nutritional plan based on the eating habits of our ancestors between 2.5 million and 10,000 years ago, living as hunter–gatherers.

Palpitations: The perceived abnormality of the heartbeat characterized by awareness of cardiac muscle contractions in the chest: hard, fast and/or irregular beats.

Pancreas: An organ located behind the stomach. It functions as part of the endocrine system and plays a role in producing several hormones (e.g., insulin). It makes and stores insulin.

Pancreatic lipase inhibitor: Lipase inhibitors are substances used to reduce the activity of lipases found in the intestine. Lipases are secreted by the pancreas when fat is present.

Pancreatitis: Inflammation of the pancreas.

Paresthesias: An abnormal sensation, typically tingling or pricking ("pins and needles"), caused chiefly by pressure on or damage to peripheral nerves.

pH: Also known as "potential of hydrogen." It indicates how alkaline or acidic a substance or solution is. Acidic substances have lower pH, whereas alkaline ones have a higher pH.

Pharmacotherapy: Drug therapy.

Phendimetrazine: A short-term supplement to diet and exercise in the treatment of obesity.

Phenotype: The set of observable characteristics of an individual resulting from the interaction of its genotype with the environment.

Phenteramine: A psychostimulant drug of the substituted amphetamine chemical class, with pharmacology similar to amphetamine. It is used medically as an appetite suppressant for short-term use, as an adjunct to exercise and reducing calorie intake.

Physical therapist: Health-care providers who help patients recover from injuries and illnesses regain movement and manage pain.

Physiological: Relating to the branch of biology that deals with the normal functions of living organisms and their parts.

Pickwickian syndrome: *See* obesity hypoventilation syndrome.

Placebo: An inactive drug that resembles a study drug (used in studies to compare the outcomes between placebo-treated groups and study-drug-treated groups).

Placebo-controlled studies: A way of testing a medical therapy in which, in addition to a group of subjects that receives the treatment to be evaluated, a separate control group receives a sham "placebo" treatment which is specifically designed to have no real effect.

Plaque: When referring to a cholesterol plaque, these can cause blockages in blood vessels and lead to decreased blood flow.

Plate method: A meal plan that suggests filling half of the plate with two servings of non-starchy vegetables, one-quarter with lean meat (3 ounces, cooked) or other high-protein food, and one-quarter with a starchy vegetable or whole-grain serving (amount varies depending on food selected).

Podagra: A medical term referring to gout of the big toe.

Polycystic ovarian syndrome (PCOS): An endocrine condition involving numerous cysts in the ovaries.

Polysomnogram (PSG): A sleep study that helps diagnose whether a sleep disorder might be present.

Post-operative: The period following an operation.

Prader-Willi syndrome: A complex genetic condition that affects many parts of the body. In infancy, this condition is characterized by weak muscle tone (hypotonia), feeding difficulties, poor growth, and delayed development.

Pre-diabetes: A condition in which a person has elevated blood sugar levels but not yet to the point of being diagnosed with type 2 diabetes. It is important because it indicates an increased risk of developing diabetes.

Pre-operative: The period before an operation.

Primary-care physician: A general medicine physician.

Pritikin principle: A very low-fat, high-carbohydrate eating plan. The focus is to eat vegetables, fruits, and high-fiber grains, based on the theory of eating low-fat, low-calorie, plant-based foods to promote weight loss and improve or prevent heart disease.

Prohormone convertase-1 deficiency (PCSK-1): A lack of prohormone convertase, prohormone convertase 3, or neuroendocrine convertase 1 and often abbreviated as PC1/3. An enzyme that in humans is encoded by the *PCSK1* gene.

Pro-opiomelanocortin (POMC) brain cells: In the brain, neurons in the arcuate nucleus express POMC mRNA that is identical to that of the pituitary. In these neurons, POMC serves as a precursor to brain β-endorphin, α-MSH, and other peptides, which have important brain functions, including a major role in energy homeostasis.

Pro-opiomalanocortin (POMC) mutation: POMC gene mutations that cause POMC deficiency result in production of an abnormally short version of the POMC protein or no protein at all.

Proprioceptive exercise: Proprioceptive and balance exercises teach your body to control the position of a deficient or an injured joint. A common example of a proprioceptive or balance exercise is the use of a balance or wobble-board after an ankle sprain.

Proton-pump inhibitors (PPIs): A class of medications used to treat acid reflux; it works by reducing the production of stomach acid.

Psychiatrist: A physician who specializes in the treatment of mental illnesses, such as major depressive disorder ("depression") or anxiety disorders.

Psychoanalytic therapy: A humanistic approach to psychotherapy that focuses on identifying the root cause of a problem.

Psychological evaluation: A way of assessing an individual's behavior, personality, cognitive abilities, and several other domains.

Psychologist: A mental-health professional (PhD or PsyD) whose focus is on the diagnosis and treatment of mental illness. In contrast to psychiatrists, psychologists typically focus on behavioral interventions, and they cannot usually prescribe medications.

Psychosis: A severe mental disorder in which thought and emotions are so impaired that contact is lost with external reality.

Psychosocial functioning: Functioning related to mental disorders and/or social problems (e.g., problems with personal relationships, work, or school).

Psychostimulants: Drugs that can improve your ability both physically and mentally during such activities. The most commonly used psychostimulants are caffeine, nicotine, amphetamines, and methamphetamine.

Psychotherapy: One of a variety of types of talking therapy.

Pulmonary arteries: The blood vessels that carry blood from the right ventricle of the heart to the lungs for oxygenation, before it is pumped to the rest of the body.

Pulmonary embolism (PE): A blood clot in an artery in the lungs. These blood clots most commonly originate from the deep veins of the legs.

Pulmonary function tests (PFTs): A group of tests that measure how well your lungs work. This includes how well you're able to breathe and how effective your lungs are able to bring oxygen to the rest of your body.

Pulmonary hypertension: High blood pressure that affects the arteries in your lungs and the right side of the heart.

Random blood glucose: A blood glucose test done regardless of the last time you ate food. Normal levels usually range from 79 mg/dl to 160 mg/dl.

Randomized controlled trial (RCT): A type of study in which one treatment is randomly assigned to a research participant and a second treatment is assigned to another participant.

Recommended dietary allowance (RDA): The average daily level of intake sufficient to meet the nutrient requirements of nearly all (97%–98%) healthy people.

Registered dietitian: A specialist in nutrition and dietary guidelines.

Reproductive endocrinologist: Endocrinologists who specialize in matters related to infertility.

Residency training programs: Residency is a period of advanced training for doctors after graduating from medical school.

Restrictive surgery: Those operations most often used for producing weight loss. Food intake is restricted by creating a small pouch at the top of the stomach where the food enters from the esophagus. The pouch initially holds about 1 ounce of food and expands to 2 to 3 ounces with time.

Risk factors: Factors that can predispose one to illness.

Roux-en-Y gastric bypass: A type of weight-loss surgery.

Selective serotonin re-uptake inhibitors (SSRIs): A class of drugs that are typically used as antidepressants in the treatment of major depressive disorder and anxiety disorders. The exact mechanism of action of SSRIs is unknown.

Septic arthritis: Also known as infectious arthritis, caused by an infectious agent (such as a bacteria) that enters the joints and causes inflammation. It is a serious condition and requires prompt treatment.

Serotonin: A compound present in blood platelets and serum that constricts the blood vessels and acts as a neurotransmitter.

Serotonin receptors: A group of G protein-coupled receptor and ligand-gated ion channels found in the central and peripheral nervous systems. They mediate both excitatory and inhibitory neurotransmission.

Serotonin syndrome: A group of symptoms that may occur following use of certain serotonergic medications or drugs. Symptoms include high body temperature, agitation, increased reflexes, tremor, sweating, dilated pupils, and diarrhea.

Set-point: The desired or target value for an essential variable, or process value of a system.

Single nucleotide polymorphism (SNPs): The most common type of genetic variation among people; a variation of a single nucleotide that occurs at a specific position in the genome.

Sleep apnea: *See* apnea.

Sleeve gastrectomy: A surgical procedure that induces weight loss by restricting food intake and stimulating hormonal changes between the brain and gut; it involves removing part of the stomach and making it smaller.

Slim-fast plan: A diet based on using meal replacements as diet aids.

Social worker: A professional concerned with helping individuals, families, groups and communities to enhance their individual and collective well-being.

Socioeconomic status: An economic and sociological combined total measure of a person's work experience and of an individual's or family's economic and social position in relation to others, based on income, education, and occupation.

Sodium channels: Channels that transmit depolarizing impulses rapidly throughout cells and cell networks, thereby enabling coordination of higher processes ranging from locomotion to cognition.

South Beach diet: A diet plan that involves eating lots of vegetables, fish, eggs, dairy, lean protein (like chicken and turkey), whole grains, and nuts. The diet is lower in carbohydrates and higher in protein and healthy fats than the typical American diet.

Statin: A type of medication that inhibits an enzyme called HMG-CoA reductase, and thereby lowers levels of circulating lipids.

Stenosis: The narrowing of a blood vessel.

Stevens-Johnson syndrome: A rare, serious disorder of your skin and mucous membranes. It's usually a reaction to a medication or an infection. Often, it begins with flu-like symptoms, followed by a painful red or purplish rash that spreads and blisters.

Stigma: A mark of disgrace associated with a particular circumstance, quality, or person.

Stress incontinence: A condition involving involuntary loss of urine with physical activity that increases intra-abdominal pressure (e.g., coughing, laughing, sneezing, lifting, exercising, bending).

Stress test: A test done to evaluate the strength of the heart and cardiovascular capacity. It is done by monitoring heart rate during increasingly strenuous exercises.

Stricture: A restriction on a person or activity (e.g., intestinal strictures are essentially narrowings in the intestine that can make it difficult for food matter to pass through).

Stroke: A neurological event caused by a lack of blood flow to a territory of the brain, usually due to a blood clot; it can cause temporary or permanent brain injury. *FAST* (*F*ace drooping, *A*rm weakness, *S*peech difficulty, *T*ime to call 9-1-1) developed to help people detect stroke, given that prompt recognition and medical care can help improve stroke outcome.

Sympathetic nervous system: Part of the autonomic nervous system (ANS), which also includes the parasympathetic nervous system (PNS). The sympathetic nervous system activates what is often termed the *fight-or-flight* response.

Sympathomimetic: Producing physiological effects characteristic of the sympathetic nervous system by promoting the stimulation of sympathetic nerves.

Synapse: A junction between two nerve cells, consisting of a minute gap across which impulses pass by diffusion of a neurotransmitter.

Syndromic obesity: A condition used to describe children and adults with obesity and cognitive delay, dysmorphic features, organ-specific features, and hyperphagia.

Systolic blood pressure: The blood pressure number written on top of a standard blood pressure reading. It measures the blood pressure in your blood vessels when your heart beats.

Thermogenic agents: Agents that stimulate the nervous system and contribute to fat loss through production of heat through metabolic stimulation.

Thiamine: Also known as thiamin or vitamin B1, this is a vitamin found in food and used as a dietary supplement. As a supplement it is used to treat and prevent thiamine deficiency and disorders that result from it, including beriberi, Korsakoff's syndrome, and Korsakoff's psychosis.

Thromboembolic disease: Problems caused by the formation of a blood clot that breaks off and leads to blockage of another (generally smaller) vessel.

Thromboembolism: The act of obstructing a blood vessel by a blood clot.

Thyroid stimulating hormone (TSH): A pituitary hormone that stimulates the thyroid gland to produce thyroxine (T_4) and then triiodothyronine (T_3), which stimulates the metabolism of almost every tissue in the body.

Topirimate: A drug approved by the US Food and Drug Administration (FDA) in combination with phentermine for weight loss.

Torsades de pointes: A specific form of polymorphic ventricular tachycardia in patients with a long QT interval. It is characterized by rapid, irregular QRS complexes, which appear to be twisting around the ECG baseline. This arrhythmia may cease spontaneously or degenerate into ventricular fibrillation.

Triglycerides: A fatty chemical found in the blood. Often elevated in type 2 diabetes, especially with poor glycemic control or high-fat diet.

Twelve-Step method: A support program utilized by Overeaters Anonymous.

Twin studies: Studies that are conducted on identical or fraternal twins to reveal the importance of environmental and genetic influences for traits, phenotypes, and disorders.

Type 2 diabetes: A type of diabetes in which a high blood glucose (sugar) is associated with insulin resistance and lack of insulin.

Uterus: Also known as the "womb," this is where the fetus develops during pregnancy.

Venous thromboembolism (VTE): A general term for any blood clot that starts in a vein. It includes both deep vein thrombosis and pulmonary embolism.

Ventilator: A device that helps assist breathing in those who are unable to do so on their own.

Vertical sleeve gastrectomy: A type of weight-loss surgery.

Visceral fat: Body fat (visceral adiposity) that is stored within the abdominal cavity and is therefore stored around a number of important internal organs; for example, the liver, pancreas, and intestines.

Vitamin B12: A water-soluble vitamin that plays essential roles in red blood cell formation, cell metabolism, nerve function and the production of DNA. Food sources of vitamin B12 include poultry, meat, fish and dairy products.

Vitamin D: A group of fat-soluble secosteroids responsible for increasing intestinal absorption of calcium, magnesium, and phosphate, and multiple other biological effects.

Waist-to-hip ratio (WHR): The dimensional ration of the circumference of the waist to that of the hips.

Weight cycling: Yo-yo dieting; in reference to the cyclical loss and gain of weight, resembling the up and down motion of a yo-yo.

Weight-loss surgery: Bariatric surgery; a variety of procedures performed on people who have obesity, achieved by reducing the size of the stomach with a gastric band, or through removal of a portion of the stomach or by resecting or rerouting the small intestine to a small stomach pouch.

Weight Watchers diet: A program that assigns every food and beverage a SmartPoints value, based on its nutrition (higher amounts of saturated fat and sugar increase the point value; higher amounts of protein bring the point value down). Choices that fill you up the longest "cost" the least, and nutritionally dense foods cost less than empty calories.

Whole30 diet: A restrictive dietary program that promises to "change your life" in 30 days through some tough-love nutritional changes. These include: no dairy, no grains, no added sugar, no alcohol, and no legumes.

Withdrawal seizures: A set of symptoms that can occur following a reduction in alcohol or other sedative-hypnotics use after a period of excessive use. Symptoms typically include anxiety, shakiness, sweating, vomiting, fast heart rate, and a mild fever.

Xanthomas: A deposition of yellowish material that is high in cholesterol, which can appear anywhere on the body, and is secondary to high levels of lipids in the body.

Xanthelasmas: When yellowish material, that is high in fat/cholesterol, deposits on the eyelid.

Yoga: A relaxation therapy.

Yo-Yo dieting: Weight cycling, in which individuals repeatedly engage in a pattern of losing weight for a period, then regaining the weight back, or gaining back even more weight.

Zone diet: A low-carbohydrate fad diet that specifies the consumption of calories from carbohydrates and protein in a specified ratio, recommending eating five times a day to make a sense of satiety that discourages overeating.

Zonisamide: A medication used to treat the symptoms of epilepsy and Parkinson's disease.

REFERENCES

1. https://asmbs.org/wp/uploads/2014/05/PsychPreSurgicalAssessment.pdf.

2. www.aafp.org/test/fpcomp/FP-E_425/pt3-s2.html.

3. https://asmbs.org/resources/long-term-survival-benefit-after-metabolic-and-bariatric-surgery.

4. https://doi.org/10.1161/CIRCULATIONAHA.111.039453 Circulation. 2012; 125: 1157–1170.

5. http://www.heart.org/HEARTORG/HealthyLiving/PhysicalActivity/FitnessBasics/American-Heart-Association-Recommendations-for-Physical-Activity-in-Adults_UCM_307976_Article.jsp#.WRUMgPnyuM8.

6. https://www.nhlbi.nih.gov/health/health-topics/topics/phys/recommend.

7. http://www.acsm.org/about-acsm/media-room/news-releases/2011/08/01/acsm-issues-new-recommendations-on-quantity-and-quality-of-exercise.

8. https://www.ncbi.nlm.nih.gov/pmc/articles/PMC3096271/).

9. http://ajcn.nutrition.org/content/87/4/801.full).

10. http://healthyamericans.org/assets/files/TFAH-2017-ObesityReport-FINAL.pdf.

11. https://www.ncbi.nlm.nih.gov/pmc/articles/PMC3005642/, accessed July 19, 2017.

12. https://www.ncbi.nlm.nih.gov/pubmed/17890752, accessed July 5, 2017.

13. https://en.wikipedia.org/wiki/Body_mass_index, accessed July 5, 2017.

14. http://www.livestrong.com/article/426250-acsm-body-fat-guidelines/, accessed July 19, 2017.

15. https://www.ncbi.nlm.nih.gov/pmc/articles/PMC3005642/, accessed July 19, 2017.

16. https://www.cdc.gov/dhdsp/data_statistics/fact_sheets/fs_heart_failure.htm.

17. The Harvard T.H. Chan School of Public Health: Deciphering media stories on diet. 2017; retrieved from https://www.hsph.harvard.edu/nutritionsource/media/.

18. The Certification Board for Obesity Educators: The certified obesity educator program. 2007; retrieved from http://www.obesityeducator.org/images/stories/CBOE_Docs/cboe-certified_obesity_counselor_program_2012.pdf.

19. Commission on Dietetic Registration: CDR's new interdisciplinary certification in obesity and weight management. 2017; retrieved from https://www.cdrnet.org/interdisciplinary.

20. Harvard University, T.H. Chan School of Public Health: The obesity prevention source. Retrieved October 29, 2017, from https://www.hsph.harvard.edu/obesity-prevention-source/.

21. The Obesity Action Coalition: Understanding your weight loss options. 2017; retrieved from http://www.obesityaction.org/educational-resources/brochures-and-guides/understanding-your-weight-loss-options-brochure.

22. Gee M, Kushner R: Does that really work? Deciphering popular weight loss trends. [webinar] 2017; retrieved from http://www.obesityaction.org/educational-resources/oac-educational-webinars.

23. US National Library of Medicine: Evaluating health information. 2017; retrieved from https://medlineplus.gov/evaluatinghealthinformation.html.

24. Agency for Healthcare Research and Quality (AHRQ): Statistical Brief #23. Bariatric surgery utilization and outcomes in 1998 and 2004. 2007; accessed October 2013 from http://www.hcup-us.ahrq.gov/reports/statbriefs/sb23.jsp.

25. American Academy of Sleep Medicine (AASM): http://www.aasmnet.org/.

26. American College of Gastroenterology (ACG): https://gi.org/.

27. American College of Rheumatology: https://www.rheumatology.org/.

28. American College of Surgeons: Metabolic and bariatric surgery accreditation and Quality improvement program (MBSAQIP®). 2017; retrieved from https://www.facs.org/quality-programs/mbsaqip.

29. American Diabetes Association: http://www.diabetes.org/.

30. American Gastroenterology Association: http://www.gastro.org/.

31. American Heart Association (AHA): http://www.heart.org/HEARTORG/.

32. American Psychological Association: Psychotherapy: understanding group therapy. Retrieved May 24, 2017, from http://www.apa.org/helpcenter/group-therapy.aspx.

33. American Psychological Association: Understanding psychotherapy and how it works. Retrieved May 24, 2017, from http://www.apa.org/helpcenter/understanding-psychotherapy.aspx.

34. American Society for Metabolic and Bariatric Surgery (ASMBS): Sleeve gastrectomy as bariatric procedure. Retrieved May 2012, from https://asmbs.org/resources/sleeve-gastrectomy-as-a-bariatric-procedure.

35. American Stroke Association: http://www.strokeassociation.org/STROKEORG/.

36. American Thoracic Society: https://www.thoracic.org.

37. Barry D, Petry NM: Obesity and psychiatric disorders. *Psychiatric Times.* 2009; 1–4. Retrieved from http://www.psychiatrictimes.com/anxiety/obesity-and-psychiatric-disorders.

38. Careers and Educational Requirements. Retrieved August 1, 2017, from http://www.psychologyschoolguide.net/social-work-careers/case-manager/.

39. Childhood and Adolescent Obesity – ASMBS Learning Center. (n.d.). Retrieved from https://asmbs.org/patients/adolescent-obesity.

40. Connelley S, Stegemann L: Who's in control? The science behind willpower. [webinar] Retrieved October 28, 2017, from http://www.obesityaction.org/educational-resources/oac-educational-webinars.

41. Gastrointestinal Surgery for Severe Obesity. NIH consensus statement online. 1991 March 25–27; 9(1): 1–20. https://consensus.nih.gov/1991/1991gisurgeryobesity084html.htm.

42. Gastrogirl: https://gastrogirl.com/.

43. Gentleman A: How psychology can beat obesity. | Society | *The Guardian.* February 19, 2013; retrieved from https://www.theguardian.com/society/2013/feb/19/patient-stomach-psychology-obesity.

44. Liquid-filled Intragastric Balloon Systems: Letter to Healthcare Providers Potential Risks. Feb 9, 2017 and Aug 10, 2017. https://www.fda.gov/Safety/MedWatch/SafetyInformation/SafetyAlertsforHumanMedicalProducts/ucm570916.htm.

45. *Massachusetts General Hospital:* Obesity medicine and nutrition fellowship. Retrieved October 28th, 2017 from http://www.massgeneral.org/digestive/assets/pdf/weight-center-two-year-fellowship.pdf.

46.   National Cancer Institute: https://www.cancer.gov/.

47.   National Heart, Lung, and Blood Institute (NHLBI): https://www.nhlbi.nih.gov/.

48.   National Stroke Association: http://www.stroke.org/.

49.   NIH: Learn About Clinical Studies. 2017a, January 2017; retrieved from https://clinicaltrials.gov/ct2/about-studies/learn – Where.

50.   NIH: NIH clinical research trials and you, the basics. 2017b, 6/21/2017; retrieved from https://www.nih.gov/health-information/nih-clinical-research-trials-you/basics.

51.   NutrtionED: Distinguishing between dietitian vs nutritionist. 2017; retrieved from https://www.nutritioned.org/dietitian-vs-nutritionist.html.

52.   Obesity Medicine Association – Clinical Leaders in Obesity Medicine. (n.d.). Retrieved from http://obesitymedicine.org.

53.   Obesity Medicine. (n.d.). In: Wikipedia. Retrieved October 28, 2017 from https://en.wikipedia.org/wiki/Obesity_medicine.

54.   Rheumatology Nurses Society (RNS): http://rnsnurse.org/.

55.   The Obesity Society: Mission & Vision. 2017; retrieved from http://www.obesity.org/about/mission-vision.

56.   The Obesity Society Task Force: Potential contributors to obesity. 2015; accessed September 19, 2017 from http://www.obesity.org/obesity/resources/facts-about-obesity/infographics/potential-contributors-to-obesity.

57.   Rubino D, Soleymani T, Kahan S: Medications for weight loss. [PDF] 2017; retrieved from http://www.obesity.org/publications/obesity-journal/patient-pages.

58.   Saunders K, Kahan S: How much weight do I need to lose? [PDF] 2017; retrieved from http://www.obesity.org/publications/obesity-journal/patient-pages.

59.   Talwalker A, McCarty F: Characteristics of physician office visits for obesity by adults aged 20 and over: United States, 2012. *NCHS Data Brief No.* 2016; 237. retrieved from https://www.cdc.gov/nchs/products/databriefs/db237.htm.

60.   Walters A. (2017): Getting Your Weight Under Control: How Psychologist Help with Weight Loss. Retrieved from: http://www.apa.org/helpcenter/weight-control.pdf.

61.   Weight Bias & Stigma>Media. http://www.uconnruddcenter.org/weight-bias-stigma-media, accessed on 5/28/2017.

62. What Is Psychiatry? (n.d.). Retrieved from https://www.psychiatry.org/patients-families/what-is-psychiatry.

63. Who is a Candidate for Bariatric Surgery? – American Society for Metabolic and Bariatric Surgery. (n.d.). Retrieved from https://asmbs.org/patients/who-is-a-candidate-for-bariatric-surgery.

64. Health.usnews.com.

65. Webmd.

66. Mayoclinic.

67. Individual diet websites.

68. How to Become a Licensed Clinical Social Worker (LCSW)? (n.d.). Retrieved from http://www.psychologyschoolguide.net/social-work-careers/how-to-become-a-clinical-social-worker/.

69. Myers A, Rosen JC.: Obesity stigmatization and coping: Relation to mental health symptoms, body image, and self-esteem. *International Journal of Obesity*. 1999; 23: 221–230.

70. Alberga AS, Pickering BJ, Alix Hayden K, et al: The role of weight teasing and weight bias internalization in psychological functioning: a prospective study among school-aged children. *European Hild & Adolescent Psychiatry*. 2017.

71. Alberts HJ, Thewissen R, Raes L: Dealing with problematic eating behaviour. The effects of a mindfulness-based intervention on eating behaviour, food cravings, dichotomous thinking and body image concern. *Appetite*. 2012; 58(3): 847–851.

72. Alciati A, Caldirola D, Grassi M, et al: Mediation effect of recent loss events on weight gain in obese people who experienced childhood parental death or separation. *Journal of Health Psychology*. 2017; 22: 101–110.

73. Allison KC, Lundgren JD, Wadden TA: Overcoming weight bias in the management of patients with diabetes and obesity. *Clinical Diabetes: A Publication of the American Diabetes Association*. 2016; 34(1): 44–50.

74. Alvarez J, Pavao J, Baumrind N, et al: The relationship between child abuse and adult obesity among California women. *American Journal of Preventive Medicine*. 2007; 33: 28–33.

75. American Association of Clinical Endocrinologists Medical Guidelines for the Clinical Use of Dietary Supplements and Nutraceuticals. *Endocrine Practice*. 2003; 9(5)417–470. https://doi.org/10.4158/EP.9.5.417.

76.   American Psychiatric Association: *Diagnostic and Statistical Manual of Mental Disorders.* 5th ed. Washington, DC: American Psychiatric Association; 2013.

77.   Anderin C, Gustafsson UO, Heijbel N, et al: Weight loss before bariatric surgery and postoperative complications: data from the Scandinavian Obesity Registry (SOReg). *Annals of Surgery.* 2015 May; 261(5): 909–913. doi: 10.1097/SLA.0000000000000839. PubMed PMID: 25211265. (n.d.).

78.   Anderson PM: Parental employment, family routines and childhood obesity. *Economics and Human Biology.* 2012; 10: 340–351.

79.   Apovian CM, Aronne LJ, Bessesen DH, et al: Pharmacological management of obesity: An endocrine society clinical practice guideline, *The Journal of Clinical Endocrinology & Metabolism.* 2015; 100(2) 342–362. https://doi.org/10.1210/jc.2014-3415.

80.   Bäckhed F: Changes in intestinal microflora in obesity: cause or consequence? *Journal of Pediatric Gastroenterology and Nutrition.* 2009; S56–S57.

81.   Baker TK, Smith GS, Jacobs NN, et al: Weight bias reduction in health professionals: a systematic review. *Clinical Obesity.* 2016; 6(3): 175–188.

82.   Basile J, Bloch MJ: Overview of hypertension in adults. In: Post T, ed. *UpToDate.* Waltham, MA: UpToDate; 2016. www.uptodate.com.

83.   Bayon VE: Sleep debt and obesity. *Annals of Medicine.* 2014; 264–272.

84.   Becker MA: Clinical manifestations and diagnosis of gout. In: Post T, ed. *UpToDate.* Waltham, MA: UpToDate; 2016. www.uptodate.com.

85.   Belle SH, Berk PD, Chapman W, et al: Baseline characteristics of participants in the Longitudinal Assessment of Bariatric Surgery-2 (LABS-2) study. *Surgery for Obesity and Related Diseases.* 2013; 9: 926. PMID: 23602493.

86.   Bellentani S, Scaglioni F, Marino M, et al: Epidemiology of non-alcoholic fatty liver disease. *Digestive Diseases.* 2010; 28(1): 155–161.

87.   Billes SK, Sinnayah P, Cowley MA: Naltrexone/Bupropion for obesity: An investigational combination pharmacotherapy for weight loss. *Pharmacological Research.* 2014; 84: 1–11.

88.   Bishop SR, Lau M, Shapiro S, et al: Mindfulness: A proposed operational definition. *Clinical Psychology: Science and Practice.* 2004; 11(3): 230–241.

89.   Blackburn GL, Greenberg I, MacNamara A, et al: The multidisciplinary approach to weight loss: defining the roles of the necessary providers. *Bariatric Times*. 2008; retrieved from bariatrictimes.com/the-multidisciplinary-approach-to-weight-loss-defining-the-roles-of-the-necessary-providers/.

90.   Block JP, DeSalvo KB, Fisher WP: Are physicians equipped to address the obesity epidemic? Knowledge and attitudes of internal medicine residents. *Preventive Medicine*. 2003; 36 (6): 669–675.

91.   Boff RM, Liboni RPA, Batista IPA, et al: Weight loss interventions for overweight and obese adolescents: a systematic review. *Eating and Weight Disorders*. 2017; 22(2): 211–229. doi: 10.1007/s40519-016-0309-1.

92.   Bolckman R, Himpens J: Long-term outcome of the laparoscopic biliopancreatic diversion with duodenal switch. *Annals of Surgery*. 2016; 264(6): 1029–1037.

93.   Borges ME: Artificially sweetened beverages and the response to the global obesity crisis. *PLoS Medicine*. 2017.

94.   Bothwell L, Greene J, Poldalsky S, et al: Assessing the gold standard: Lessons learned from the history of RCTs. *New England Journal of Medicine*. 2016; 374: 2175–2181.

95.   Botta RA: Television images and adolescent girls' body image disturbance. *Journal of Communication*. 1999; 49(2): 22–41.

96.   Boulos R, Vikre EK, Oppenheimer S, et al: ObesiTV: How television is influencing the obesity epidemic. *Physiol Behav*. 2012; 107(1): 146–153.

97.   Bray GA, Ryan DH: Update on obesity pharmacotherapy. *Annals of the New York Academy of Science*. 2014; 1311: 1–13.

98.   Britannica TE: Adipose cell. 2015; retrieved from *Encyclopædia Britannica*. https://www.britannica.com/science/adipose-cell.

99.   Brownell KD: *Weight Bias: Nature, Consequences, and Remedies*. New York: Guilford Press; 2005.

100. Brownell KD, Rodin J: Medical, metabolic, and psychological effects of weight cycling. *Archives of Internal Medicine*. 1994; 154(12): 1325–1330.

101. Burgermaster ME: Exploring the role of sugar-sweetened beverage consumption in obesity among New Yorkers using propensity score matching. *Journal. Academy of Nutrition and Dietetics*. 2017; 753–762.

102. Butsch WS: Obesity medications: what does the future look like? *Current Opinions in Endocrinology Diabetes Obesity.* 2015; 22(5): 360–366. doi: 10.1097/med.0000000000000192.

103. Carels RA, Hinman NG, Burmeister JM, et al: Weight bias in graduate school admissions. *Obesity.* Silver Spring, Md: 2013; 21(5): 918–920.

104. Carr D, Friedman MA: Body weight and the quality of interpersonal relationships. *Social Psychology Quarterly.* 2006; 69: 127–149.

105. Carr D, Friedman MA: Is obesity stigmatizing? Body weight, perceived discrimination, and psychological well-being in the United States. *Journal of Health and Social Behavior.* 2005; 46: 244–259.

106. Cefalu WT, Bray GA, Home PD, et al: Advances in the science, treatment, and prevention of the disease of obesity: Reflections from a diabetes care editors' expert forum. *Diabetes Care.* 2015; 38(8): 1567–1582.

107. Centers for Disease Control and Prevention (CDC): Age-adjusted percent distributions (with standard errors) of participation in leisure-time aerobic and muscle-strengthening activities that meet the 2008 federal. *Summary Health Statistics: National Health Interview Survey.* Center for Disease Control and Prevention. 2014.

108. Centers for Disease Control and Prevention (CDC): *Heart Disease Facts.* Available at https://www.cdc.gov/heartdisease/facts.htm, accessed June 12, 2017.

109. Centers for Disease Control and Prevention (CDC): *Stroke Facts.* Available at https://www.cdc.gov/stroke/facts.htm, accessed June 6, 2017.

110. Chiba T, Tsuchiya T, Komatsu T, et al: Development of calorie restriction mimetics as therapeutics for obesity, diabetes, inflammatory and neurodegenerative diseases. *Current Genomics.* 2010; 11(8): 562–567. http://doi.org/10.2174/138920210793360934.

111. Choi HK, Atkinson K, Karlson EW: Obesity, weight change, hypertension, diuretic use, and risk of gout in men. *Archives in Internal Medicine.* 2005; 165(7): 742–748.

112. Christakis NA, Fowler JH: The spread of obesity in a large social network over 32 years. *New England Journal of Medicine.* 2007; 357: 370–379.

113. Chronic Hypertension. Stanfordhealthcare.org. https://stanfordhealthcare.org/medical-conditions/blood-heart-circulation/chronic-hypertension.html, accessed September 2017.

114. Chwastiak L, Tek C: Management of obesity in the psychiatrist's office. *World Psychiatry.* 2014; 13(2): 193–195. doi: 10.1002/wps.20138.

115. Claussnitzer M, et al: FTO obesity variant circuitry and adipocyte browning in humans. *New England Journal of Medicine*. 2015; 373(10): 895–907.

116. Cohen A: Big fat stereotypes play out on the small screen. Transcript of *Morning Edition*. National Public Radio, aired 8/8/2011.

117. Corella D, Ordovas JM: Can genotype be used to tailor treatment of obesity? State of the art and guidelines for future studies and applications. *Minerva Endocrinol*. 2013; 38(3): 219–235.

118. Crandall CS, D'Anello S, Sakalli N, et al: An attribution-value model of prejudice: Anti-fat attitudes in six nations. *Personality and Social Psychology Bulletin*. 2001; 27(1): 30–37.

119. Cruwys T, Bevelander KE, Hermans RCJ: Social modeling of eating: A review of when and why social influence affects food intake and choice. *Appetite*. 2015; 86: 3–18.

120. Cummings SM, Pratt JSA, Kaplan LM: Evaluation and management of obesity. In: Carlson K, Eisenstat S, eds. *Primary Care of Women*. 2nd ed. New York: Mosby–Year Book. 2002; pp 238–249.

121. Dalen J, Smith BW, Shelley BM, et al: Pilot study: Mindful Eating and Living (MEAL): weight, eating behavior, and psychological outcomes associated with a mindfulness-based intervention for people with obesity. *Complementary Therapies in Medicine*. 2010; 18(6): 260–264.

122. D'Argenio A, Mazzi C, Pecchioli L, et al: Early trauma and adult obesity: Is psychological dysfunction the mediating mechanism? *Physiology & Behavior*. 2009; 98: 543–546.

123. Daubenmier J, Kristeller J, Hecht FM, et al: Mindfulness intervention for stress eating to reduce cortisol and abdominal fat among overweight and obese women: an exploratory randomized controlled study. *Journal of Obesity*. 2011.

124. Definition & Facts for GER & GERD: Niddk.nih.gov. https://www.niddk.nih.gov/health-information/digestive-diseases/acid-reflux-ger-gerd-adults/definition-facts, accessed September 2017.

125. Derosa G, Maffioli P, Sahebkar A: Improvement of plasma adiponectin, leptin and C-reactive protein concentrations by orlistat: a systematic review and meta-analysis. *British Journal of Clinical Pharmacology*. 2016; 81(5): 819–834. http://doi.org/10.1111/bcp.12874.

126. Deurenberg P, Weststrate J, Seidell J: Body mass index as a measure of body fatness: Age- and sex-specific prediction formulas. *British Journal of Nutrition*. 1991; 65 (2): 105–114. doi: 10.1079/BJN19910073.

127. Devine CE: "Pizza is cheaper than salad": assessing workers' views for an environmental food intervention. *Obesity*. 2007; 15.

128. Dhurandhar EA: The aetiology of obesity beyond eating more and exercising less. *Best Practice & Research Clinical Gastroenterology*. 2014; 533–544.

129. Digital in 2017: Global overview. Retrieved September 2017, from We are social. https://wearesocial.com/special-reports/digital-in-2017-global-overview. 2017.

130. Diabetes. Cdc.gov. https://www.cdc.gov/media/presskits/aahd/diabetes.pdf, accessed September 2017.

131. Dixon JB, Dixon ME, O'Brien PE: Depression in association with severe obesity: changes with weight loss. *Archives of Internal Medicine*. 2003; 163(17): 2058–2065.

132. Dokken BAS: The physiology of body weight regulation: are we too efficient for our own good? *Diabetes Spectrum*. 2007; 166–170.

133. Driesbach S: Weight stereotyping: The secret way people are judging you based on your body. In. *Glamour*. 2012.

134. Dua S, Bhuker M, Sharma P, et al: Body mass index relates to blood pressure among adults. *North American Journal of Medical Science*. 2014; 6(2): 89–95.

135. Ducharme J: Mass General study finds a new way to use poop pills. Researchers may have identified a safer, more effective type of capsule. *Boston Magazine*. 2016.

136. Durso LE, Latner JD, Ciao AC: Changes in weight bias and perceived employability following weight loss and gain. *Obesity Surgery*. 2015; 25(3): 568–570.

137. Eckel RH, Kahn SE, Ferrannini E, et al: Obesity and type 2 diabetes: What can be unified and what needs to be individualized? *Journal of Clinical Endocrinology and Metabolism*. 2011; 96(6): 1654–1663.

138. Epstein LH, Wrotniak BH: Future directions for pediatric obesity treatment. *Obesity (Silver Spring)*. 2010; 18 Suppl 1: S8-12. doi: 10.1038/oby.2009.425.

139. El-Hadi M, Birch DW, Gill RS, et al: The effect of bariatric surgery on gastroesophageal reflux disease. *Canadian Journal of Surgery*. 2014; 57(2): 139–144.

140. El-Serag H: The association between obesity and GERD: A review of the epidemiological evidence. *Digestive Diseases and Science*. 2008; 53(9): 2307–2312.

141. El-Serag HB, Sweet S, Winchester CC, et al: Update on the epidemiology of gastroesophageal reflux disease: a systematic review. *Gut.* 2014 Jun; 63(6): 871–880.

142. Esteghamati A, Mazaheri T, Vahidi Rad M, et al: Complementary and alternative medicine for the treatment of obesity: A critical review. *International Journal of Endocrinology and Metabolism.* 2015; 13(2): e19678. http://doi.org/10.5812/ijem.19678

143. Everhart JE, Ruhl CE: Burden of digestive diseases in the United States Part III: Liver, biliary tract, and pancreas. *Gastroenterology.* 2009 Apr; 136(4): 1134–1144.

144. Exline JJ, Zell AL, Bratslavsky E, et al: People-pleasing through eating: Sociotropy predicts greater eating in response to perceived social pressure. *Journal of Social and Clinical Psychology.* 2012; 31: 169.

145. Fabricatore AN, Crerand CE, Wadden TA, et al: *Obesity Surgery.* 2006; 16: 567. https://doi.org/10.1381/096089206776944986.

146. Fabbrini E, Sullivan S, Klein S: Obesity and nonalcoholic fatty liver disease: Biochemical, metabolic and clinical implications. *Hepatology.* 2010; 51(2): 679–689.

147. Fakhouri TH: Physical activity in U.S. youth aged 12–15 years, 2012. *NCHS Data Brief.* Centers for Disease Control and Prevention. 2014.

148. Farias MA: Set-point theory and obesity. *Metabolic Syndrome and Related Disorders.* 2011; 85–89.

149. Fava M: Weight gain and antidepressants. *The Journal of Clinical Psychiatry.* 1999; 61: 37–41.

150. Fawcett KA, Barroso I. The genetics of obesity: FTO leads the way. *Trends in Genetics.* 2010; 26 (6): 266–274.

151. Flegal KE: Trends in obesity among adults in the United States, 2005 to 2014. *Journal of the American Medical Association.* 2016; 2284–2291.

152. Foster GD, Makris AP, Bailer BA: Behavioral treatment of obesity. *The American Journal of Clinical Nutrition.* 2005; 82(1): 230S–235S.

153. Franco ME: Availability of healthy foods and dietary patterns: The multi-ethnic study of atherosclerosis. *The American Journal of Clinical Nutrition.* 2009; 897–904.

154. Fresno M, Alvarez R, Cuesta N: Toll-like receptors, inflammation, metabolism and obesity. *Archives of Physiology and Biochemistry.* 2011; 117: 151–164.

155. Friedman JM, Halaas JL: Leptin and the regulation of body weight in mammals. *Nature*. 1998; 395: 763–770.

156. Friedman KE, Reichmann SK, Costanzo PR, et al: Weight stigmatization and ideological beliefs: relation to psychological functioning in obese adults. *Obesity research*. 2005; 13: 907–916.

157. Fryar CD, Carroll MD, Ogden CL: Prevalence of overweight, obesity, and extreme obesity among adults aged 20 and over: United States, 1960–1962 through 2013–2017. *National Center for Health Statistics.*

158. Fryar CD, Chen TC, Li X: Prevalence of uncontrolled risk factors for cardiovascular disease: United States, 1999–2010. *NCHS Data Brief.* 2012; 103: 1–8.

159. Gadde KM, Pritham Raj Y: Pharmacotherapy of obesity: Clinical trials to clinical practice. *Current Diabetes Reports*. 2017; 17(5): 34. doi: 10.1007/s11892-017-0859-2.

160. Gagner M: Is Sleeve gastrectomy always an absolute contraindication in patients with Barrett's? *Obesity Surgery*. 2016 Apr; 26(4): 715–717. doi: 10.1007/s11695-015-1983-1.

161. Galic S, Oakhill JS, Steinberg GR: Adipose tissue as an endocrine organ. *Mol Cell Endocrinology* 2010; 316: 129–139.

162. Gangwisch JE: Inadequate sleep as a risk factor for obesity: analyses of the NHANES I. *Sleep*. 2005; 1289–1296.

163. Germer C: What is mindfulness. *Insight Journal*. 2004; 22: 24–29.

164. Gill RS, Birch DW, Shi X, et al: Sleeve gastrectomy and type 2 diabetes mellitus: a systematic review. *Surgery for Obesity and Related Diseases*. 2010 Nov-Dec; 6(6): 707–713.

165. Giordano S, Victorzon M: The impact of preoperative weight loss before laparoscopic gastric bypass. *Obesity Surgery*. 2014 May; 24(5): 669–674. doi: 10.1007/s11695-013-1165-y. PubMed PMID: 24357128. (n.d.).

166. Gobel CH, Tronnier VM, Munte TF: Brain stimulation in obesity. *International Journal of Obesity*. London: 2017; doi: 10.1038/ijo.2017.150.

167. Goodman E, Whitaker RC: A prospective study of the role of depression in the development and persistence of adolescent obesity. *Pediatrics*. 2002; 110(3): 497–504.

168. Gortmaker SL, Must A, Sobol AM, et al: Television viewing as a cause of increasing obesity among children in the United States, 1986–1990. *Archives of Pediatric and Adolescent Medicine* 1996; 150: 356–362.

169. Greenberg BS, Eastin M, Hofschire L, et al: Portrayals of overweight and obese individuals on commercial television. *American Journal of Public Health*. 2003; 93(8): 1342–1348.

170. Gregory Traversy JPC: Alcohol consumption and obesity: An update. *Current Obesity Reports*. 2015; 122–130.

171. Groesz LM, McCoy S, Carl J, et al: What is eating you? Stress and the drive to eat. *Appetite*. 2012; 58(2): 717–721.

172. Guarino B: Google faulted for racial bias in image search results for black teenagers. *Washington Post*. 6/10/16, 2016.

173. Guidelines for Media Portrayals of Individuals Affected by Obesity. http://www.uconnruddcenter.org/resources/upload/docs/what/bias/media/MediaGuidelines_PortrayalObese.pdf, accessed 5/28/2107.

174. Gujral H, Tea C, Sheridan M: The effects of reality television on weight bias: an examination of The Biggest Loser. *Obesity (Silver Spring, Md)*. 2012; 20(5): 993–998.

175. Haidich A: Meta-analysis in medical research. *Hippokratia*. 2010; 14 (Suppl 1): 29–37.

176. Hassan Y, Head V, Jacob D, et al: Lifestyle interventions for weight loss in adults with severe obesity: a systematic review. *Clinical Obesity*. 2016; 6(6): 395–403. doi: 10.1111/cob.12161.

177. Heart Disease Facts. Cdc.gov. https://www.cdc.gov/heartdisease/facts.htm, accessed September 2017.

178. Himmelstein MS, Puhl RM, Quinn DM: Intersectionality: An understudied framework for addressing weight stigma. *American Journal of Preventive Medicine*. 2017.

179. Himpens J, Dobbeleir J, Peeters G: Long-term results of laparoscopic sleeve gastrectomy for obesity. *Annals of Surgery*. 2010 Aug; 252 (2): 319–324.

180. Holland S, Dallos R, Olver L: An exploration of young women's experiences of living with excess weight. *Clinical Child Psychology and Psychiatry*. 2012; 2011; 17: 538.

181. Hottman JM, Helmick CG, Hannan CJ, et al: Prevalence of obesity among adults with arthritis—United States, 2003–2009. *Morbidity and Mortality Weekly Report*. 2011; 60(16): 509–513.

182. Hubner C, Baldofski S, Zenger M, et al: Ethnic identity and implicit anti-fat bias: Similarities and differences between African-American and Caucasian women. *Ethnicity & Disease*. 2016; 26(1): 69–76.

183. Hwang KO, Ottenbacher AJ, Green AP, et al: Social support in an Internet weight loss community. *International Journal of Medical Informatics*. 2010; 79(1): 5–13.

184. Hypertension in the United States. Stateofobesity.org. http://stateofobesity.org/hypertension/, accessed September 2017.

185. Jackson SE, Kirschbaum C, Steptoe A: Hair cortisol and adiposity in a population-based sample of 2,527 men and women aged 54 to 87 years. *Obesity*. 2017; 25(3): 539–544.

186. Jaremka LM, Belury MA, Andridge RR, et al: Novel links between troubled marriages and appetite regulation: Marital distress, ghrelin, and diet quality. *Clinical Psychological Science*. 2016; 4: 363–375.

187. Jensen MD, Ryan DH, Apovian CM, et al: 2013 AHA/ACC/TOS guideline for the management of overweight and obesity in adults: A report of the American College of Cardiology/American Heart Association Task Force on practice guidelines and the obesity society. *Circulation*. 2014; 129: S102.

188. Johns DJ, Hartmann-Boyce J, Jebb SA, et al: Diet or exercise interventions vs. combined behavioral weight management programs: a systematic review and meta-analysis of direct comparisons. *Journal of the Academy of Nutrition and Dietetics*. 2014; 114(10): 1557–1568.

189. Kahn BA: Obesity and insulin resistance. *The Journal of Clinical Investigation*. 2000; 473–481.

190. Kahn SE, Hull RL, Utzschneider KM: Mechanisms linking obesity to insulin resistance and type 2 diabetes. *Nature*. 2006; 444: 840–846.

191. Kahrilas PJL: Medical management of gastroesophageal reflux disease in adults. In: Post T, ed. *UpToDate*. Waltham, MA: UpToDate; 2016. www.uptodate.com.

192. Kane A: How fat affects arthritis. Arthritis.org. http://www.arthritis.org/living-with-arthritis/comorbidities/obesity-arthritis/fat-and-arthritis.php, accessed September 2017.

193. Karine ST: Sleep curtailment in healthy young men is associated with decreased leptin levels, elevated ghrelin levels, and increased hunger and appetite. *American College of Physicians*. 2004; 846–850.

194. Kass AE, Wildes JE, Coccaro EF: Identification and regulation of emotions in adults of varying weight statuses. *Journal of Health Psychology*. 2017; 1359105316689604.

195. Kenchaiah S, Evans JC, Levy D, et al: Obesity and the risk of heart failure. *New England Journal of Medicine*. 2002; 347: 305–313.

196. Key Statistics for Endometrial Cancer? Cancer.org. https://www.cancer.org/cancer/endometrial-cancer/about/key-statistics.html, accessed September 2017.

197. Kim SH, Chun HJ, Choi HS, et al: Current status of intra-gastric balloon for obesity treatment. *World Journal of Gastroenterology*. 2016 Jun 28; 22(24): 5495–5504. Published online 2016 Jun 28.

198. Kimbro RT, Brooks-Gunn J, McLanahan S: Racial and ethnic differentials in overweight and obesity among 3-year-old children. *American Journal of Public Health*. 2007; 97: 298–305.

199. King WC, Chen JY, Courcoulas AP, et al: Alcohol and other substance use after bariatric surgery: Prospective evidence from a US multicenter cohort study. *Surgery for Obesity and Related Diseases*. Author manuscript; available in PMC 2018 Aug 1.

200. Kodama K, Noda S, et al: Depressive disorders as psychiatric complications after obesity surgery. *Psychiatry Clinical Neuroscience*. 1998; 52(5): 471–476.

201. Kristeller JL, Wolever RQ: Mindfulness-based eating awareness training for treating binge eating disorder: the conceptual foundation. *Eating Disorders*. 2010; 19(1): 49–61.

202. Kuo CF, Grainge MJ, Zhang W, et al: Global epidemiology of gout: prevalence, incidence and risk factors. *Nature Reviews Rheumatology*. 2015; 11:649–662.

203. Ladenheim EE: Liraglutide and obesity: a review of the data so far. *Drug Design, Development and Therapy*. 2015; 9: 1867–1875. http://doi.org/10.2147/DDDT. S58459Redman LM & Ravussin E. (2010).

204. Latner JD, Rosewall JK, Simmonds MB: Childhood obesity stigma: association with television, videogame, and magazine exposure. *Body Image*. 2007; 4: 147–155.

205. Le MH, Devaki P, Ha NB, et al: Prevalence of non-alcoholic fatty liver disease and risk factors for advanced fibrosis and mortality in the United States. *PLOS One*. 2017; 12(3): 1–13.

206. LeMont D, Reto CS, Ritz SJ: (2004). assessmentpsychology.com.

207. Livingstone KM: FTO genotype and weight loss: systematic review and meta-analysis of 9563 individual participant data from eight randomised controlled trials. *BMJ*. 2016.

208. Lo B, Field M: (2009) *Conflicts of interest in medical research, education, & practice*. Washington D.C. National Academies Press.

209. Locke AE, et al: Genetic studies of body mass index yield new insights for obesity biology. *Nature*. 2015; 518 (7538):197–206.

210. Lonneman DJ, Rey JA, McKee BD: Phentermine/topiramate extended-release capsules (Qsymia) for weight loss. *Pharmacy and Therapeutics*. 2013; 38(8): 446–452.

211. Lopes EA: Short-term metabolic changes and de novo lipogenesis induced by a high-carbohydrate meal in lean and obese subjects. *Proceedings of the Nutrition Society*. 2000.

212. Lopez-Velazquez JA, Silva-Vidal KV, Ponciano-Rodriguez G, et al: The prevalence of nonalcoholic fatty liver disease in the Americas. *Annals of Hepatology*. 2014; 13(2): 166–178.

213. Lorcaserin for the treatment of obesity. *Drugs of Today*. Barcelona, Spain: 1998; 46(12): 901–910. http://doi.org/10.1358/dot.2010.46.12.1556433.

214. Lumeng JC, Chervin RD: Epidemiology of pediatric obstructive sleep apnea. *Proceedings of the American Thoracic Society*. 2008 Feb 15;5(2): 242–252.

215. Lunagariya NA, Patel NK, Jagtap SC, Bhutani KK: Inhibitors of pancreatic lipase: state of the art and clinical perspectives. *EXCLI Journal*. 2014; 13: 897–921.

216. Luppino FS, de Wit LM, Bouvy PF, et al: Overweight, obesity, and depression: a systematic review and meta-analysis of longitudinal studies. *Archives of General Psychiatry*. 2010; 67(3): 220–229.

217. Macht M, Simons G: Emotions and eating in everyday life. *Appetite*. 2000; 35(1): 65–71.

218. Mahoney NA, El Mourabet M, Weyant K: Bariatric surgery and inflammatory bowel disease [AGA abstract 306]. *Gastroenterology*. 2011;140 (5 Supp): S792.

219. Managing Diabetes. Joslin.org. http://www.joslin.org/info/managing-diabetes.html, accessed September 2017.

220. Marks JW: GERD (Acid Reflux, Heartburn). Medicinenet.com. http://www.medicinenet.com/gastroesophageal_reflux_disease_gerd/article.htm, accessed September 2017.

221. Martin JA: Births: Final data for 2015. *National Vital Statistics Report*. 2017.

222. Martinez J: Body-weight regulation: causes of obesity. *Proceedings of the Nutrition Society*. 2000; 337–345.

223. McElroy SL, Kotwal R, Malhotra S, et al: Are mood disorders and obesity related? A review for the mental health professional. *J of Clinical Psychiatry*. 2004; 65(5): 634–651.

224. McFadden KM: Cross-addiction: From morbid obesity to substance abuse. *Bariatric Nursing and Surgical Patient Care.* June 2010, 5(2): 145–178.

225. Merai R, Siegel C, Rakotz M, et al: CDC grand rounds: A public health approach to detect and control hypertension. *Morbidity and Mortality Weekly Report.* 2016 Nov 18; 65(45): 1261–1264. Available at: https://www.cdc.gov/bloodpressure/index.htm.

226. Misra M: Obesity pharmacotherapy: Current perspectives and future directions. *Current Cardiology Reviews.* 2013; 9(1): 33–54. http://doi.org/10.2174/157340313805076322.

227. Mitchell NS, Ellison MC, Hill JO, et al: Evaluation of the effectiveness of making Weight Watchers available to Tennessee Medicaid (TennCare) recipients. *Journal of General Internal Medicine.* 2013; 28(1): 12–17.

228. Modave F, Shokar NK, Peñaranda E, et al: Analysis of the accuracy of weight loss information search engine results on the internet. *American Journal of Public Health.* 2014; 104(10): 1971–1978.

229. Müller MJ, Bosy-Westphal A, Heymsfield SB: Is there evidence for a set point that regulates human body weight? F1000 Med Rep. 2010; 2: 59. Published online 2010 Aug 9. doi: 10.3410/M2-59.

230. Müller MJ, Enderle J, Bosy-Westphal A: Changes in energy expenditure with weight gain and weight loss in humans. *Current Obesity Reports.* 2016; 5(4): 413–423. doi: 10.1007/s13679-016-0237-4.

231. Myers A, Rosen JC: Obesity stigmatization and coping: relation to mental health symptoms, body image, and self-esteem. *International Journal of Obesity.* 1999; 23(3): 221–230.

232. Nandagopal R, Brown RJ, Rother KI: Resolution of type 2 diabetes following bariatric surgery: Implications for adults and adolescents. *Diabetes Technology Therapy.* 2010 Aug; 12(8): 671–677.

233. National Center for Chronic Disease Prevention and Health Promotion, Centers for Disease Control and Prevention, National Diabetes Statistics Report, 2014. Available at https://www.cdc.gov/diabetes/pdfs/data/2014-report-estimates-of-diabetes-and-its-burden-in-the-united-states.pdf. Accessed June 14, 2017.

234. National Institutes of Health (U.S.), National Institute of Diabetes and Digestive and Kidney Diseases (U.S.), National Heart, Lung, and Blood Institute, National Center for Biotechnology Information (U.S.). *Clinical Guidelines on the Identification, Evaluation, and Treatment of Overweight and Obesity in Adults: The Evidence Report.* Vol no. 98-4083; no. 98-4083. Bethesda, MD: National Heart, Lung, and Blood Institute in cooperation with the National Institute of Diabetes and Digestive and Kidney Diseases; 1998.

235. Neves DBDJ, Caldas ED: Determination of caffeine and identification of undeclared substances in dietary supplements and caffeine dietary exposure assessment. *Food and Chemical Toxicology.* 2017 Jul;105: 194–202. doi: 10.1016/j.fct.2017.03.063. (2003).

236. Obesity Rates & Trends Overview. Stateofobesity.org. https://stateofobesity.org/obesity-rates-trends-overview/ Accessed September 2017.

237. O'Brien PE, Dixon JB, Brown W: The laparoscopic adjustable gastric band (Lap-Band): a prospective study of medium-term effects on weight, health and quality of life. *Obesity Surgery.* 2002; 12(5): 652–660.

238. O'Brien PE, MacDonald L, Anderson M, et al: Long-term outcomes after bariatric surgery: fifteen-year follow-up of adjustable gastric banding and a systematic review of the bariatric surgical literature. *Annals of Surgery.* 2013 Jan; 257(1): 87–94.

239. Olson KL, Emery CF: Mindfulness and weight loss: a systematic review. *Psychosomatic Medicine.* 2015; 77(1): 59–67.

240. Omalu BI, Ives DG, Buhari AM, et al: Death rates and causes of death after bariatric surgery for Pennsylvania Residents, 1995 to 2004. *Archives of Surgery.* 2007; 142(10): 923–928. doi: 10.1001/archsurg.142.10.923.

241. Ozier AD, Kendrick OW, Knol LL, et al: The eating and appraisal due to emotions and stress (EADES) questionnaire: Development and validation. *Journal of the American Dietetic Association.* 2007; 107(4): 619–628.

242. Pantenburg B, Sikorski C, Luppa M, et al: Are medical students aware of their anti-obesity bias? *Academic Medicine: Journal of the Association of American Medical Colleges.* 2013; 88(7): 978–982.

243. Paxton SJ, Damiano SR: Weight bias: A systematic review of characteristics and psychometric properties of self-report questionnaires. *Obesity Facts.* 2017; 10(3): 223–237.

244. Perusse L, et al: The human obesity gene map: the 2004 update. *Obesity Research.* 2005; 13 (3): 381–490.

245. Pesa JA, Syre TR, Jones E: Psychosocial differences associated with body weight among female adolescents: the importance of body image. *Journal of Adolescent Health*. 2000; 26(5): 330–337.

246. Peterson CM, Thomas DM, Blackburn GL, et al: Universal equation for estimating ideal body weight and body weight at any BMI. *American Journal of Clinical Nutrition*. 2016 May; 103(5): 1197–1203. Published online 2016 Mar 30.

247. Petry NM, Barry D, Pietrzak RH, et al: Overweight and obesity are associated with psychiatric disorders: Results from the National Epidemiologic Survey on alcohol and related conditions. *Psychosomatic Medicine*. 2008; 70(3): 288–297.

248. Phelan SM, Burgess DJ, Yeazel MW, et al: Visual portrayals of obesity in health media: promoting exercise without perpetuating weight bias. *Health Education Research*. 2015; 30(4): 580–590.

249. Phelan SM, Puhl RM, Burke SE, et al: Impact of weight bias and stigma on quality of care and outcomes for patients with obesity. *Obesity Reviews: An Official Journal of the International Association for the Study of Obesity*. 2015; 16(4): 319–326.

250. Picolo ME: Harris-Benedict equation and resting energy expenditure estimates in critically ill ventilator patients. *American Journal of Critical Care*. 2016; e21–e29.

251. Plaxe SC, Mundt AJ: Overview of endometrial carcinoma. In: Post T, ed. *UpToDate*. Waltham, Mass.: UpToDate; 2016. www.uptodate.com.

252. Ponce J, Woodman G, Swain J, et al: The REDUCE pivotal trial: A prospective, randomized controlled pivotal trial of a dual intra-gastric balloon for the treatment of obesity. *Surgery for Obesity and Related Diseases*. 2015; 11 (4): 874–881.

253. Potential Contributors to Obesity Infographic. (n.d.). Retrieved September 22, 2017, from Obesity Society: http://www.obesity.org/obesity/resources/facts-about-obesity/infographics/potential-contributors-to-obesity. 2017.

254. Prosch N: *I Grow*. RetrievedSeptember 22, 2017, from Light, moderate, and vigorous activity. http://igrow.org/healthy-families/health-and-wellness/light-moderate-and-vigorous-activity/. 2013.

255. Puhl RM, Brownell KD: Confronting and coping with weight stigma: An investigation of overweight and obese adults. *Obesity*. 2006; 14(10): 1802–1815.

256. Puhl RM, Latner JD, O'Brien K, et al: The mixed impact of medical school on medical students' implicit and explicit weight bias. *Medical Education*. 2015; 49(10): 983–992.

257. Punjabi NM: The epidemiology of adult obstructive sleep apnea. *Proceedings of the American Thoracic Society*. 2008 Feb 15; 5(2): 136–143.

258. Raves DM, Brewis A, Trainer S, et al: A multinational examination of weight bias: predictors of anti-fat attitudes across four countries. *International Journal of Obesity (2005)*. 2015; 39(7): 1166–1173.

259. Reddon HJ-L: The importance of gene–environment interactions in human obesity. *Clinical Science*. 2016; 1571–1597.

260. Reinehr T, et al: Definable somatic disorders in overweight children and adolescents. *Journal of Pediatrics*. 2007; 150 (6): 618–622, 622 e1-5.

261. Ren CJ, Patterson E, Gagner M: Early results of laparoscopic biliopancreatic diversion with duodenal switch: a case series of 40 consecutive patients. *Obesity Surgery*. 2000; 10(6): 514–523, discussion 524.

262. Renjilian DA, Perri MG, Nezu AM, et al: Individual versus group therapy for obesity: Effects of matching participants to their treatment preferences. *Journal of Consulting and Clinical Psychology*. 2001; 69(4): 717.

263. Rhee K: Childhood overweight and the relationship between parent behaviors, parenting style, and family functioning. *The Annals of the American Academy of Political and Social Science*. 2008; 615: 12–37.

264. Rogers JM, Ferrari M, Mosely K, et al: Mindfulness-based interventions for adults who are overweight or obese: a meta-analysis of physical and psychological health outcomes. *Obesity Reviews*. 2017; 18(1): 51–67.

265. Romero-Corral A, Caples SM, Lopez-Jimenez F, et al: Interactions between obesity and obstructive sleep apnea. *Chest*. 2010; 137(3): 711–719.

266. Roslin MS, Cripps C, Peristeri A: Bariatric and metabolic surgery: current trends and what's to follow. *Current Opinions in Gastroenterology*. 2015; 31(6): 513–518. doi: 10.1097/mog.0000000000000223.

267. Rowston WM, McCluskey SE, Gazet JC, et al: Eating behavior, physical symptoms and psychological factors associated with weight reduction following the Scopinaro operation as modified by Gazet. *Obesity Surgery*. 1992; 2: 355–360.

268. Roza AA: The Harris Benedict equation reevaluated: Resting energy requirements and the body cell mass. *The American Journal of Clinical Nutrition*. 1984; 168–182.

269. Rudolph A, Hilbert A: Association between weight bias internalization and metabolic syndrome among treatment-seeking individuals with obesity. *Obesity (Silver Spring, Md).* 2017; 25(2): 317–322.

270. Sarkhosh K, Birch DW, Sharma A, et al: Complications associated with laparoscopic sleeve gastrectomy for morbid obesity: a surgeon's guide. *Canadian Journal of Surgery.* 2013 Oct; 56(5): 347–352. doi: 10.1503/cjs.033511.

271. Sasaki A, Nitta H, Otsuka K, et al: Bariatric surgery and non-alcoholic fatty liver disease: Current and potential future treatments. *Frontiers in Endocrinology.* 2014; 5(164): 1–6.

272. Schakel SE: Adjusting a nutrient database to improve calculation of percent calories from macronutrients. *Journal of Food Composition and Analysis.* 2009; S32–S36.

273. Schauer PR, Ikramuddin S, Gourash W, et al: Outcomes after laparoscopic Roux-en-Y gastric bypass for morbid obesity. *Annals of Surgery.* 2000; 232(4): 515–529.

274. Schmandt RE, Iglesias DA, Co NN, Lu KH: Understanding obesity and endometrial cancer risk: Opportunities for prevention. *American Journal of Obstetrics and Gynecology.* 2011; 205(6): 518–525.

275. Schneider HJ, Friedrich N, Klotsche J, et al; The predictive value of different measures of obesity for incident cardiovascular events and mortality. *The Journal of Clinical Endocrinology & Metabolism.* 2010; 95(4): 1777–1785. https://doi.org/10.1210/jc.2009-1584.

276. Schnitzer E, Goldstein L, Futterman B: (2017). Obesity and pain management. Practical Pain Management, 1-3. Retrieved from https://www.practicalpainmanagement.com/treatments/pharmacological/obesity-pain-management.

277. Schousboe KE: Sex differences in heritability of BMI: a comparative study of results from twin studies in eight countries. *Twin Research and Human Genetics.* 2003; 409–421.

278. Schumann R: Anesthesia for the obese patient. In: Post T, ed. *UpToDate.* Waltham, Mass.: UpToDate; 2016. www.uptodate.com.

279. Schvey NA, Puhl RM, Brownell KD: The impact of weight stigma on caloric consumption. *Obesity.* 2011; 19: 1957–1962.

280. Schwartz MW, Woods SC, Porte D, et al: Central nervous system control of food intake. *Nature.* 2000; 404: 661–671.

281. Scott KM, Bruffaerts R, Simon GE, et al: Obesity and mental disorders in the general population: results from the world mental health surveys. *International Journal of Obesity*. 2008; 32(1): 192–200.

282. Scott KM, McGee MA, Wells JE, et al: Obesity and mental disorders in the adult general population. *Journal of Psychosomatic Research*. 2008; 64(1): 97–105.

283. Sethi M, Chau E, Youn A, et al: Long-term outcomes after biliopancreatic diversion with and without duodenal switch: 2-, 5-, and 10-year data. *Surgery for Obesity and Related Diseases*. 2016 Nov; 12(9): 1697–1705.

284. Shah MB: Obesity and sexuality in women. *Obstetrics and Gynecology Clinics of North America*. 2009; 36: 347–360.

285. Shaw K, O'Rourke P, Del Mar C, Kenardy J. Psychological interventions for overweight or obesity. *Cochrane Database Systematic Reviews*. 2005; 2(2).

286. Shi X, Karmali S, Sharma AM: A Review of Laparoscopic Sleeve Gastrectomy for Morbid Obesity. *Obesity Surgery*. 2010; 20 (8): 1171.

287. Shu L, et al. Shared genetic regulatory networks for cardiovascular disease and type 2 diabetes in multiple populations of diverse ethnicities in the United States. *PLoS Genetics*. 2017; 13(9): e1007040.

288. Sjöström L, Narbro K, Sjöström CD, et al: Swedish Obese Subjects Study. Effects of bariatric surgery on mortality in Swedish obese subjects. *New England Journal of Medicine*. 2007; 357(8): 741–752.

289. SleepApnea.Mayoclinic.org.(2015).http://www.mayoclinic.org/diseases-conditions/sleep-apnea/basics/definition/con-20020286. Accessed September 2017.

290. Snyder EE, et al: The human obesity gene map: The 2003 update. *Obesity Research*. 2004; 12 (3): 369–439.

291. Spiel EC, Rodgers RF, Paxton SJ, et al: Toddlers' bias to look at average versus obese figures relates to maternal anti-fat prejudice. *Journal of Experimental Child Psychology*. 2016; 142: 195–202.

292. Stanford F: Obesity and breastfeeding: Exploring the relationship. *Breastfeeding Medicine*. 2016; 411–412.

293. Stein PD, Beemath A, Olson RE: Obesity as a risk factor in venous thromboembolism. *American Journal of Medicine*. 2005. 118 (9): 978–980.

294. Stice E, Presnell K, Shaw H, Rohde P: Psychological and behavioral risk factors for obesity onset in adolescent girls: A prospective study. *Journal of Consulting and Clinical Psychology.* 2005; 195–202.

295. Strategies to Prevent Obesity. Cdc.gov. https://www.cdc.gov/obesity/strategies. Accessed September 2017.

296. Strauss RS. Childhood obesity and self-esteem. *Pediatrics.* 2000; 105(1): e15–e15.

297. Strecher VJ, Seijts GH, Kok GJ, et al: Goal setting as a strategy for health behavior change. *Health Education Quarterly.* 1995; 22(2): 190–200.

298. Strine TW, Mokdad AH, Dube SR, et al: The association of depression and anxiety with obesity and unhealthy behaviors among community-dwelling US adults. *General Hospital Psychiatry.* 2008; 30(2): 127–137.

299. Strohl KP: Overview of obstructive sleep apnea in adults. In: Post T, ed. *UpToDate.* Waltham, Mass.: UpToDate; 2016. www.uptodate.com.

300. Stunkard AJ, Harris JR, Pedersen NL, et al: The body-mass index of twins who have been reared apart. *New England Journal of Medicine.* 1990; 322: 1483–1487.

301. Sucandy I, Antanavicius G, Bonanni F, Jr: Outcome analysis of early laparoscopic sleeve gastrectomy experience. *JSLS.* 2013 Oct-Dec; 17(4): 602–606.

302. Sumithran P, et al: Long-term persistence of hormonal adaptations to weight loss. *New England Journal of Medicine.* 2011; 365(17): 1597–1604.

303. Surgery for Diabetes. Asmbs.org. https://asmbs.org/patients/surgery-for-diabetes, accessed September 2017.

304. Tanneberger A, Ciupitu-Plath C: 'He's got his father's bias': Parental influence on weight bias in young children. *British Journal of Developmental Psychology.* 2016; 34(2): 198–211.

305. Tchoukalova YD: Regional differences in cellular mechanisms of adipose tissue gain with overfeeding. *Proceeding of the National Academy of Sciences of the United States of America.* 18226–18231. 2010; Retrieved from: Proceedings of the National Academy of Sciences of the United St. 2010.

306. Teasdale JD, Segal ZV: *The mindful way through depression: Freeing yourself from chronic unhappiness.* Guilford Press; 2007.

307. Thompson JK, Heinberg LJ: The media's influence on body image disturbance and eating disorders: We've reviled them, now can we rehabilitate them? *Journal of Social Issues.* 1999; 55(2): 339–353.

308. Thompson JK, Stice E: Thin-ideal internalization: Mounting evidence for a new risk factor for body-image disturbance and eating pathology. *Current Directions in Psychological Science.* 2001; 10(5): 181–183.

309. Throop EM, Skinner AC, Perrin AJ, et al: Pass the popcorn: "Obesogenic" behaviors and stigma in children's movies. *Obesity.* 2014; 22: 1694–1700.

310. Torres SJ, Nowson CA: Relationship between stress, eating behavior, and obesity. *Nutrition.* 2007; 23(11): 887–894.

311. Tsai AG, Wadden TA: Systematic review: an evaluation of major commercial weight loss programs in the United States. *Annals of Internal Medicine.* 2005; 142(1): 56–66.

312. Tucker ME: "Fat" jokes aren't funny. *Diabetes Forecast.* 2014; 1.

313. Type 2 diabetes. Thehealthsite.com. http://www.thehealthsite.com/type-2-diabetes/, accessed September 2017.

314. UCLA: Calories Count. *Student Nutrition Awareness Campaign.* 2005.

315. Van Nieuwenhove Y, Dambrauskas Z, Campillo-Soto A, et al: Preoperative very low-calorie diet and operative outcome after laparoscopic gastric bypass: a randomized multicenter study. *Archives of Surgery.* 2011 Nov; 146(11): 1300–1305. doi: 10.1001/archsurg.2011.273. PubMed PMID: 22106323. (n.d.).

316. Veldhorst MA, Noppe G, Jongejan MH, et al: Increased scalp hair cortisol concentrations in obese children. *The Journal of Clinical Endocrinology & Metabolism.* 2014; 99(1): 285–290.

317. Voisin SE: Many obesity-associated SNPs strongly associate with DNA methylation changes at proximal promoters and enhancers. *Genome Medicine.* 2015.

318. Wang Y, Wang QJ: The prevalence of prehypertension and hypertension among US adults according to the new joint national committee guidelines: new challenges of the old problem. *Archives of Internal Medicine.* 2004 Oct 25; 164(19): 2126–2134.

319. Wardle JE: Evidence for a strong genetic influence on childhood adiposity despite the force of the obesogenic environment. *The American Journal of Clinical Nutrition.* 2008; 398–404.

320. Weihs K, Fisher L, Baird M: Families, health and behavior: Families, systems & health: *The Journal of Collaborative Family Healthcare* [serial online]. Spring 2002; 20(1): 7.

321. Weinsier R: Etiology of obesity: methodological examination of the set-point theory. *Journal of Parenteral and Enteral Nutrition.* 2001; 103–110.

322. Wendelboe AM, McCumber M, Hylek EM, et al: Global public awareness of venous thromboembolism. *Journal of Thrombosis and Haemostasis*. 2015; 13(8): 1365–1371.

323. Wesdorp I, Bosman D, de Graaff A, et al: Clinical presentations and predisposing factors of cholelithiasis and sludge in children. *Journal of Pediatric Gastroenterology and Nutrition*. 2000 Oct. 31(4): 411–417.

324. What is deep vein thrombosis? Nhlbi.nih.gov. https://www.nhlbi.nih.gov/health/health-topics/topics/dvt, accessed September 2017.

325. What is diabetes? Niddk.nih.gov. https://www.niddk.nih.gov/health-information/diabetes/overview/what-is-diabetes, accessed September 2017.

326. Whitaker RC, et al: Predicting obesity in young adulthood from childhood and parental obesity. *New England Journal of Medicine*. 1997; 337 (13): 869–873.

327. White MA, Martin PD, Newton RL, et al: Mediators of Weight Loss in a Family-Based Intervention Presented over the Internet. *Obesity Research*. 2004; 12(7): 1050–1059.

328. WHO. Global Strategy on Diet, Physical Activity and Health. 2004. www.who.int/dietphysicalactivity/strategy/eb11344/strategy_english_web.pdf.

329. Wing RR, Jeffery RW: Benefits of recruiting participants with friends and increasing social support for weight loss and maintenance. *Journal of Consulting and Clinical Psychology*. 1999; 67(1): 132.

330. Wilson PWF, Douglas PS: Epidemiology of coronary heart disease. In: Post T, ed. *UpToDate*. Waltham, Mass.: UpToDate; 2016. www.uptodate.com.

331. World Health Organization, Diabetes Fact Sheet. Available at http://www.who.int/mediacentre/factsheets/fs312/en/, accessed June 15, 2017.

332. Wright SA: Causes of obesity. *Abdominal Radiology*. 2012; 730–732.

333. Wulkan ML, Walsh SM: The multi-disciplinary approach to adolescent bariatric surgery. *Seminars in Pediatric Surgery*. 2014; 23(1): 2–4. doi: 10.1053/j.sempedsurg.2013.10.012.

334. Yamamiya Y, Cash TF, Melnyk SE, et al: Women's exposure to thin-and-beautiful media images: Body image effects of media-ideal internalization and impact-reduction interventions. *Body image*. 2005; 2(1): 74–80.

335. Yang G, De Staercke C, Hooper WC: The effects of obesity on venous thromboembolism: A review. *Open Journal of Preventive Medicine*. 2012; 2(4): 499–509.

336. Yanovski SZ, Yanovski JA: Long-term drug treatment for obesity: A systematic and clinical review. *The Journal of the American Medical Association.* 2014; 311(1): 74–86. http://doi.org/10.1001/jama.2013.281361.

337. Yuen M, et al. 2016. Poster.

338. Zhang Y, Jordan JM: Epidemiology of Osteoarthritis. *Clinics in Geriatric Medicine.* 2010; 26(3): 355–369.

339. Zheng Y, Wang M, He S, et al: Short-term effects of intra-gastric balloon in association with conservative therapy on weight loss: a meta-analysis. Journal of Translational Medicine. 2015; 13: 246. Published online 2015 Jul 29.

340. Zlot A, Newell A, Silvey K, Arail K: Addressing the obesity epidemic: A genomics perspective. *Preventing Chronic Disease.* 2007; 4 (2): A31.

341. Zwickert K, Rieger E: A qualitative investigation of obese women's experiences of effective and ineffective social support for weight management. *Clinical Obesity.* 2014; 4: 277–286.

INDEX

calories, 35–36
Camellia Sinensis, 146
cancer
    associated with obesity, 77, 80–81
    as contraindication for surgery, 155
carbonic anhydrase inhibition, 141
cardiac catheterization, 58
cardiac ischemia, 144
cardiac stress test, 154
cardiorespiratory activity, 112–116, 116
cardiovascular conditions, 54–62
case-control studies, 209
case manager, 178
Centers for Disease Control and
        Prevention (CDC), 28, 114
central nervous system (CNS), 122, 139
central sleep apnea, 63
cerebrovascular accident (CVA), 58–59
cerebrovascular disease, 58–59
Certification Board of Obesity Educators,
        208
Certified Obesity Educators, 208
children and adolescents
    age when weight bias develops, 198
    bariatric surgery for, 176
    BMI categories for, 47
    cortisol levels of, 15
    depression interacting with weight gain
        in, 16
    dietary habits of family affecting, 94
    effects of your obesity on, 96, 97
    emotions of, 12
    infant health risks based on maternal
        age, 42
    infant health risks from mother's obe-
        sity, 34–35, 82
    low self-esteem in, 183
    obesity rates in, 2
    parental influence on weight bias, 198

risk of obesity as adults, 46
trauma of, affecting later obesity, 95
TV shows and movies, effects of, 27–28
type 1 diabetes in, 69
cholecystectomy, 75
cholecystitis, 75
cholecystokinin, 138
cholelithiasis (gallstones), 74–75
cholesterol levels, 7, 55, 175
chromium picolinate, 147
chromosomes, 87
circulatory system, 54, 60
cirrhosis, 76, 77, 155
clinical depression. *See* depression
clinical research trials
    considering participation in, 168, 170
    definition of, 166
    eligibility requirements for, 168
    informed consent for, 169
    location of, 169
    phases of, 167
    placebos used in, 169
    potential benefits, 167
    potential risks, 168
    results from, 171
    types of, 166
    who pays for, 169
coagulation factors, 60
cognitive-behavioral therapy (CBT),
        187–190
cognitive impairment, 155
colonoscopy, 160
comfort food, 41
co-morbidities, 7
complementary and alternative medicine
        (CAM), 145
complete blood count (CBC), 154
complex (mixed) sleep apnea, 63
computerized tomography (CT) scan, 59

Made in the USA
Monee, IL
17 January 2023

25474813R00164